Agility at Any Age

DISCOVER THE SECRET TO BALANCE, MOBILITY, AND CONFIDENCE

Mary Derbyshire

Please note the author cannot accept any responsibility for mishap or injury resulting from the practice of any of the principles, techniques and exercises set out in this book and its videos. This book and its videos are not intended as guidance for the treatment of serious health problems. Please refer to a medical professional if you are in any doubt about any aspect of your condition.

ISBN: 1540811190
ISBN 13: 9781540811196
Library of Congress Control Number: 2016920309
CreateSpace Independent Publishing Platform
North Charleston, South Carolina

For Amy

"You have been my friend," replied Charlotte. "That in itself is a tremendous thing."

—E. B. White, *Charlotte's Web*

Contents

Introduction · ix

Chapter 1   When I'm Sixty-Four ·1

Chapter 2   I Keep Holding On ·9

Chapter 3   Get Up, Stand Up ·19

Chapter 4   Stand by Me ·30

Chapter 5   Let It Be· ·39

Chapter 6   Every Breath You Take ·49

Chapter 7   Walk This Way ·55

Chapter 8   Let's Get Physical· ·63

About FM Alexander· ·77

Recommended Reading ·81

Acknowledgments ·85

About the Author· ·89

Introduction

http://mderbyshire.com/welcome-lets-get-started/

This book describes the basic first steps toward enjoying a healthy, life-changing way to move and live. I wrote it because I want to share a few of the most valuable things I have learned in my thirty years as a fitness instructor and twenty-four years as an Alexander Technique teacher, helping people who are struggling with pain and stiffness from injuries, accidents, and just plain old bad habits.

I have worked with kick-boxing champions, cellists, surfers, organists, gardeners, stroke survivors, military veterans, teenagers, moms, dads, sisters, brothers, grandparents, and a ninety-year-old harpsichordist. In the last ten years, I have worked particularly closely with seniors—both in group programs and in one-on-one sessions—and it is this group that I had in mind when I set out to write this book.

In this book, you will learn about the Alexander Technique and how this technique—coupled with range-of-motion activities—will change your life from moving with tension, stiffness, and pain to moving with improved balance, agility, and ease.

You will need a few simple things in order to get started. You will need a hard chair—preferably wooden—with a flat seat, like a kitchen chair or dining-room chair. You will need a long mirror that you can see while sitting in or standing up from your chair. You will need three or four paperback books of varying thicknesses. You will need a quiet place where you can lie down on the floor. If you cannot get up and down from the floor, you may use your bed.

One suggestion I have is that it might be fun to read this book out loud with a partner or a friend or even in a book club. The book is filled with instructions and activities to get you moving better, and I think that it would be fun to do these with another person if you are so inclined.

Finally, this book is interactive. There are two ways to view the accompanying videos. You can go to my website, www.mderbyshire.com, and view the videos there, or you can use a mobile phone or tablet that is equipped with an app called a QR (quick response) code reader. QR codes are like the bar code on items at the grocery store. All the QR codes throughout the book can be scanned with your smartphone or iPad to watch the videos that were created especially for you.

I use videos to illustrate ways to sit, stand, and move better. Each of the videos is approximately one to two minutes long and will teach you how to live with less muscular stress and tension so that you can live a happier, more active life.

How to Scan the QR Codes in This Book

Step 1. Download a free QR code reader onto your smartphone by searching the App Store. I selected the Kaywa Reader because it is free of advertisements.

Step 2. Tap the app once it has downloaded to your phone; this will open up the reader. Tap again, and your camera will appear to be on. Hover over the code you wish to scan, and the camera will automatically take a picture of the QR code; then your phone will be directed to the respective web page on www.mderbyshire.com that contains each video message.

You can find free QR code readers at the App Store for your phone or device.

CHAPTER 1

When I'm Sixty-Four

Do you wish you could turn back the clock to a time when you could move with better balance and ease? Are you convinced that aging inevitably brings stiffness and pain? Does fear of falling prevent you from enjoying the activities you love, like golf, tennis, or gardening? You know that you would feel younger if you could move more easily and with less pain and stiffness.

Everywhere you turn these days, you are told to exercise and move. We all know the benefits of exercise: exercise for a healthy heart, exercise to improve bone density, and exercise to promote brain health. But what if movement in and of itself is painful and difficult? If you have difficulty getting out of a chair, how can you ever be expected to go for a walk? If your knees hurt or your back aches and your neck is stiff, how can you be expected to move more when everything about you is telling you to move less!

This is all very real, and you are definitely not alone. I work every day with seniors who are trapped by this dilemma: the more they hurt, the less they move, and the less they move, the more they hurt. They begin to think, "This aging thing really, really stinks." They start to believe in one of the greatest lies of all time, which is this: Getting old means you are doomed to a life of pain and stiffness. Getting old means you must abandon those things that you love to do because it is too hard to physically do them.

We all have the image etched in our brains of the hobbling old granny or grandpa stooped over a cane or a walker, barely able to move. This image is false, and it is cruel. It is a preconceived idea that can become a self-fulfilling prophecy, if you are not careful.

You do not have to age that way! You can move easily into your senior years with balance and poise. You can learn how to move more freely and with an increased range of motion.

Certainly as we age, our bodies definitely change. Our eyesight and hearing may diminish, and our range of motion may decline. Our balance becomes less certain. We lose confidence in our bodies and choose to do fewer and fewer things. Fear of falling consumes many of us and forces us to opt out of a lot of activities. In my practice, this is a common observation.

The Centers for Disease Control and Prevention (CDC) says that medical costs for seniors falling down are $34 billion annually. The CDC also says that one out of three seniors falls every year. Clearly, balance and the lack thereof—falling—are an enormous problem that needs to be addressed. This book is devoted to finding those solutions.

There is a way to turn back the clock. There is a skill you can learn that will teach you how to move better so that you can function better. The principles described in this book will teach you to move more easily with less muscular tension and improved balance, mobility, and ease. You can learn this skill. It is fun, effective, and really quite easy.

http://mderbyshire.com/we-dont-move-like-we-used-to/

Think about when you were a child. Chances are, when you were young, you ran, skipped, jumped, and tumbled with no effort and certainly no pain or stiffness. How many kids, after playing outdoors for hours on end, complain about a bad back or a sore knee? None that I know of!

Have you ever stopped and asked yourself when your ability to enjoy this joyful, free-flowing movement ended? When you look around, do you notice that some people move more easily than others? Think about the people in your life. See them walking or sitting or talking and expressing themselves.

Perhaps you have friends who seem relatively healthy, yet they have difficulty walking or even sitting in a chair, while you also have friends the same age who still ride a bicycle or go hiking with their grandkids. Do you ever stop to wonder what creates this difference? Why are some people more balanced and agile than others? Perhaps it is the way in which they use their bodies.

Would you agree that we all move differently and that we all have habits? These habits, maintained over a lifetime, can interfere with our natural postural mechanisms. These habits are very often the cause of unnecessary muscular tension and pain.

You can see these habits and even identify the origins of some. You might walk like one of your parents or pick up a friend's expression or copy a gesture your spouse uses. We pick up some habits by mimicking those around us. Habits also develop after an accident or trauma. For instance, if because of an injury you wore a cast on your leg, your gait may have changed. You could develop a habit around this injury. Because high heels create poor body mechanics, women who walk in them develop bad habits.

Sometimes habits develop around badly designed furniture. Sitting on overly stuffed and cushioned sofas and chairs encourages the habit of slouching. Car seats are notorious for promoting bad sitting habits. Chairs with backward-sloping seats wreak havoc on our posture.

There are many particulars in our lives that influence habit. Habit is not only if you tilt your head to the right, slump in a chair, or have the tendency to shuffle while you walk. Habit is your tempo, intention, and energy—even your disposition. Your habits are part of you, good or bad. Some of the bad can really interfere with the way that you move and think and react in this world.

Let me emphasize this point: your bad habits are interfering with the way you were designed to move and think and be. You may think that your back is hurting you, when, in fact, it is you and your poor habits that are hurting your back.

By identifying bad habits, people can then learn how to move better with less muscular tension and greater ease. Improving their balance and increasing their mobility is the most important goal.

So we have these habits that interfere with the way we move. Most of us don't think about how we move unless we are in pain or are feeling self-conscious, and then the pain or the self-consciousness contributes to the litany of our habits.

This explains why, when you were two, three, or four years old, you moved with ease. You had an elongated back, a head poised on top of the spine, and an ability to squat and move effortlessly. No one taught you how to move. No one taught you how to crawl or walk. Walking, crawling, and smiling are inherited and hardwired through nature.

There is integrity in your structure. But by the age of four or five—just about the time when you entered school and started to feel self-con-scious—this integrity is often compromised.

The beautiful way in which the head relates to the spine begins to change. Your head is no longer balanced on top of your spine, and in-stead your head starts to fall backward off your spine. Or it may even fall forward from your spine, and you start to slump through the torso. This attitude of the head/neck/spine is part of the fight-or-flight reflex or the fear reflex.

http://mderbyshire.com/the-fear-reflex/

So, in short, we become habituated to fear. I believe that this happens in large part because at this age we start to identify less with our parents and caregivers and more with ourselves as individuals. We become self-conscious. Self-consciousness is under the umbrella of fear.

At this point, you start to become habituated to the slump, and to accommodate the slump, your body tightens and stiffens in order to maintain balance.

Your parents or your teachers probably nagged you to sit up straight, and you may have tried to sit up straight by pulling up through your torso or pulling back your shoulders and puffing up your chest, but this did not work.

Sitting like this feels strained and tight and, over a short period of time, painful. So you go back to your slouch, but this time the slouch has been piled on with all of your versions of what you think standing up straight should look like.

Then comes your adolescence and thus more self-consciousness. You contort yourself even more so that by your midteens, you don't move anything like you did as a small child. By the age of twenty, you have a bad neck or bad back; by the age of thirty, you have developed migraines; and at forty your knees are bothering you. Because you cannot get the exercise you need, you are anxious and depressed. By fifty you've decided to give up tennis or running, and by sixty you need a double-knee replacement. And all of this started because at the age of four, your head—that thirteen-pound bowling ball that is supposed to sit on top of your spine—has shifted.

Because your body will do anything in its power to prevent your head hitting the ground, your muscles have contorted and stiffened and held you together in the most ungainly way.

The key is that the way your head relates to your neck and the rest of your spine dictates how well you function. This, in part, is what Frederick Matthias Alexander (FM) observed back in the late eighteen hundreds and is the primary principle of his teaching called the Alexander Technique (AT).

All human beings respond to a fearful situation in the same way. We shorten and contract the muscles in the back of our necks and in our backs so that the head is pulled backward and down off the spine. Our heart rate and thus our pulse increases. The blood rushes from our arms and legs and goes to our center. Our digestion slows down, and our breathing becomes shallower. Our palms and feet sweat. Our bodies go into red alert, and we are ready to fight, flee, freeze, or succumb. The problem is that many of us become conditioned to this fearful response and cannot get out of it. Thus, the way our heads relate to our spines becomes habituated with the fight-or-flight response. It is very stressful for us to be in constant fight-or-flight mode.

The principles taught in this book will give you the tools to stop this constant stress and will teach you to move and think with less hardship and improved resiliency.

Before we go any further, let's rethink exercise. Every day we are told to exercise. Exercise for health. Go for a walk. Go for a run. Ride your bike. Swim. Dance. Move. Get moving—because when you exercise, all sorts of wonderful physiological and psychological changes occur.

The benefits of exercise are enormous. But for most of us, exercise is a chore. For most, the word *exercise* takes on a bad connotation. To me, it implies a codified way to move, a certain prescription of a right and wrong way to do things. To me, exercise feels as if it is removed from you in some way and not part of your natural expression.

There are exercise experts and exercise science; there are exercise fads and exercise gurus. There is a whole culture of exercise. But here is the thing: exercise is just movement, and humans are designed to move. We are a lot like sharks that must move to breathe and stay alive. We, too, need to move to maintain health (Vlahos 2011).

There is extensive research into the harm of a sedentary lifestyle. We do great harm to ourselves by sitting too much. We need to move more. But there are other demoralizing aspects of our current social-fitness culture.

One of these aspects is what I call the militarization of fitness—the boot-camp classes and their imitations that supposedly make you so fit that you could go off to war! Few of us need to be that fit! This whole idea of no pain, no gain as the best indicator for a good workout is just plain wrong. We are beating ourselves up.

The first question that needs to be asked is, fit for what? What do you want to be fit for? If you want to run a marathon, then you need to train for a marathon, but if you want to be more balanced and more mobile, then balance and mobility is what you need to explore.

If you were to go into a gym or health club, you would see a room full of machines that promote cardiovascular health: StairMasters and ellipticals, stationary bikes, and maybe a rowing machine. In another section, you would find dozens of pieces of equipment for strength training: barbells, dumbbells, benches, and the really big machines like Nautilus and Cybex that let you sit and lift weights. We have all these machines costing thousands of dollars to replicate what you could achieve by lifting a three-pound dumbbell that costs seven dollars. And adding to the absurdity, there is nothing to address balance, mobility, and agility, except maybe a yoga class or two that, by the way, in many places is taught like that boot-camp fitness class. There is a lot of research out there that supports my claims (Reynolds 2012, 1–24).

My question is, why can't all of this be kinder and more holistic?

This book will teach you how to make the transition from the drudg-ery of exercise to a joyful exploration of movement. The book is divided into seven lessons. Each lesson is a chapter. So now you are my student! Welcome to my teaching studio—this book!

Chapter 8, "Let's Get Physical," brings together all you have learned into a fun series of movement sequences that will open your range of motion, challenge and improve your balance, and just make you feel great!

Proceed through the book as it is laid out. Do not skip ahead. I would suggest reading and practicing one lesson a day or every few days or even a week. Do all of the activities in each lesson or chapter, and continue to practice what you have learned daily. Remember, knowledge without ap-plication has no relevance. In order for you to change, your body needs to repeat the new experience over and over again. To be well is to move well, and to move well is to move with balance, freedom, and ease.

CHAPTER 2

I Keep Holding On

You cannot be who you are not. Simply
rest, sit still, and unknot.
—ANA CLAUDIA ANTUNES, *THE DAO WORKBOOK*

et us start with an activity that you do all day long and probably don't give much attention to—sitting. Yes, sitting is an activity and a great place to start to learn how to move more easily. In this chapter you will learn several basic steps to follow that will make sitting upright easier. The age-old reprimand of "sit up straight" will seem outdated and useless. Let's learn how to sit well!

Most people want "good posture," and most people think that to sit and stand well takes a lot of discipline and physical strength. Nothing could be further from the truth.

But before we learn to sit well, let's sit poorly. Take your hard chair (remember in the introduction, I mentioned that you will need a hard chair, like a kitchen chair or a dining-room chair, and a mirror), and place your mirror nearby so that you can observe yourself. Take a seat. Notice how you are sitting. Where are you making contact with the chair? Where are your feet? Are you comfortable? Can you sit like this awhile?

If you are not already slouching, then slouch now. What is this like? What do you notice? Can you feel compression in your torso? What do you think is happening to your lungs, your stomach, your intestines, and your other organs when you are sitting like this and all of your weight is compressing them? How can your body function properly when you are slouching and pulled down like this? How can you breathe well and digest well when you are so compressed?

Now do the opposite. Try to sit up straight just like your mother or your teacher always told you to do. Let's follow the conventional instructions of how to get "good" posture. Pull your shoulders back. Lift your chest. Suck in your stomach. Now breathe in. Most likely, you cannot breathe deeply. And most likely after a couple of minutes, you cannot maintain this posture or position. So not only can you not breathe easily, but your back, shoulders, and neck are starting to cramp up. Clearly this does not work. It is not a lack of willpower. Correcting your posture like this is impossible.

Let's learn a new way to improve your sitting. I call this lesson your Guided Sitting Practice. Sit toward the edge of the chair, and slide your palms underneath your bum. Make sure that your palms are facing toward the sky and the backs of your hands are on the seat of the chair. Do you feel the bony bits under your hands? Everyone, no matter what bum size, can feel these bony bits. These are your sitz bones or, to be anatomically correct, your ischial tuberosities, and if you sit on them, you will automatically sit up taller. Now slide your hands out.

The bottom of the pelvis is shaped like a U. You need to sit on the bottom of the U. Most of us rock to the back of the U, and this forces us to slump. Or we rock to the front of the U, and then we arch and hyperextend our lower backs. You can play with this by rocking back and forth on your pelvis. See how your relationship with the chair and where it supports you under your pelvis affects the relationship of your head and your spine! So all those people who have told you for years to sit up straight and to pull your shoulders back were wrong. They should have been asking you to sit on your sitz bones!

http://mderbyshire.com/**foot-placement**/

Next, place your feet underneath you. Most of us have a tendency to place the feet too far forward, which forces us to rock back off our sitz bones toward our sacrum or lower back, and then we must haul ourselves forward over our feet in order to stand up. Or else we pull our legs back far under the chair, which puts a lot of unnecessary strain on our hamstrings—the muscles in the back of the thigh. Your feet need to be underneath you, just a little bit behind the knee. It does not matter if your heels touch the floor, just so long as some part of the foot is touching the floor.

http://mderbyshire.com/your-head-and-your-spine/

Here is a little anatomy lesson. Place your finger just in front of your ears and your thumb just at the notch behind your earlobe and gently nod your head up and down. In from here is where your head and spine articulate. It is called the atlanto-occipital (AO) joint. If you ask most people where their head and their neck meet, they will point to a spot just below the back of the skull. Because the spine is remarkably flexible, the head is able to move from there, but it is not a joint or a place of articulation.

There are thirty-three vertebrae in the spinal column: seven vertebrae in the cervical region of the spine called your neck, twelve vertebrae in the thoracic spine (think of your rib cage), five in the lumbar spine, often referred to as your lower back, and four in the coccygeal region. There are five verte- brae in the sacral spine, but these become fused when we reach adulthood. Although your spine has many moving parts, it likes to move in one piece.

Now go back to the area in front of your ears and temple and behind the earlobe. Gently nod your head yes, and then gently shake your head no. When we say yes, we are nodding our head at C1 (first cervical vertebra) or the atlas, and when we say no, we are moving from C2 (second cervical vertebra) or the axis.

Oftentimes the way that we think about ourselves anatomically is how we actually move. If we can correct our misconceptions about how the body moves, it can help us move better. This is the concept behind Body Mapping. You can learn more about Body Mapping here at www.bodymap.org.

Before we go any further, let's talk about the concept of *use*. How you use yourself is how you move, think, and react. We will apply this word as a verb as in, "Let's discuss how well you use yourself." And as a noun as in, "She has good use." When we refer to it as a noun, pronounce *use* to rhyme with *loose*. Essentially this entire book is about teaching you how to use yourself in a better way. Better use creates better functioning. When you use yourself well and your functioning improves, your movement will be- come better balanced and easier.

So now it is time to think about how you use yourself. Notice yourself sitting on the chair. Your feet are underneath you. Some part of your foot is on the floor. Your head is articulating at the AO joint. Your spine is between your pelvis and your head. You are not doing anything; you are just noticing without any judgment how you are sitting.

I want you to think. Just think of your spine releasing toward your head. Think of your head lightly and easily resting on top of your spine at the place we just identified as the AO joint. Do not try to sit up straight. This is very different from trying to sit up "straight" or with "good" posture.

Practicing sitting in this way brings about better posture, but we are not striving for it. Our goal is to think about ourselves in a new and constructive way, and as a result we improve posture, mobility, and balance.

Here is the key: when you let go of unnecessary muscular tension, you move more easily. Your habits almost always manifest themselves through muscular tension and muscular contraction. We respond to pretty much everything, whether it is emotional, physical, psychological, or spiritual, with muscular tension and contraction. Our muscles can do one of two things: they can contract or not contract. Most often when we are stimulated in any way, our muscles respond by contracting.

So we are consciously deciding to release unnecessary tension and not to contract. Instead, we let go and expand ourselves into the situation. You are not trying to do anything. Do not try; do not do. Just be.

Allow yourself to sit on your sitz bones. Allow your feet to be underneath you. Allow your head to be on the top of your spine. Allow your spine to release toward the head. Now think about your neck. Just think the thought of softening your neck. It sounds funny, I know, but just tell yourself, "I will not tighten my neck."

http://mderbyshire.com/let-me-clarify-forward/

When you start to let go of unnecessary tension in your neck, your nose may drop slightly downward, and your head may rock slightly forward. If you place your hand on your forehead at about the place we called the third eye, this is what we mean by forward. You are not jutting your head forward; it is just the intention of your head to be forward rather than backward.

The reason the head rocks forward is because the front of the head is heavier than the back of the head. So when you let go of the contracted muscles in the neck, the head releases forward, and the nose slightly moves down. I cannot say the following enough. This is not a "doing." This is a thinking and an allowing.

Are you starting to understand that you are creating the problem? The good news is that if you are creating the problem, you can learn how to stop it. That is what the technique is about: stopping your habits of poor use so that you can move the way you were meant to.

Let's come back to your Guided Sitting Practice. You are sitting on a hard chair. You are sitting on your sitz bones. Your feet are underneath you. You are thinking of allowing your head to release at your AO joint. You are thinking of allowing your spine to spring up in the direction of your head. You are thinking this; you are not trying to pull your spine up, nor are you trying to sit up straight. No trying allowed!

Our practice is thinking, not *doing* or *trying*. We bring about change through our thinking and through our attention to ourselves in ways that we have never done before.

Now I want you to think about softening your tongue. Think about softening your jaw. Think about softening your neck. All the while, you are thinking of your head resting on the top of the spine.

You are learning a new and constructive way to think about yourself. Most likely before now you may not have had a constructive way to think about yourself. Perhaps before now, your most common thoughts about yourself typically fell into the categories of, "Am I too short, or am I too tall? Am I too fat, or am I too thin? I should be sitting up straight. Why do I slouch?" Your new way of thinking is your change agent.

You have not been asked to do anything. You have not been told to improve your sitting by doing one hundred sit-ups or five-minute planks. You have not been told to strengthen your core. Instead, you have been asked to think about yourself differently. We can bring about physical and emotional change just by thinking of ourselves in a different way. The body and mind are one. You are a whole person. One. Alexander coined the term *psychophysical* to describe this unity. When we affect the physical, we affect the mind, and when we affect the mind, we affect the physical.

The power of our conscious mind is astonishing. Our job is to take our unconscious habits and bring them to a conscious level. The tricky thing is that our habits are mostly unconscious. We have no idea what our habits are. You know that experience of seeing your reflection in a window, and you think, "Yikes, is that me?" We have no idea how we really are.

http://mderbyshire.com/**weird-and-different/**

Here is a fun way for you to experience the force of habit and how pernicious it is. Lace your fingers together. Notice how this feels. Now take your hands apart and relace them, but this time move your fingers one finger over. How does that feel? Weird! It feels funny. It feels wrong. It feels funny and wrong because you have the habit of lacing them the first way. When I asked you to lace your fingers, you automatically laced them in your habitual way. The first way of lacing your fingers feels right. This habit feels good. This habit feels comfortable. But is the second way of lacing your fingers wrong? No, of course not. The second way of lacing your fingers isn't wrong. It just FEELS wrong.

I call this the Weird and Different experience, or WD for short. Alexander called it *faulty sensory appreciation*. You would never lace your fingers the second way unless you stopped and consciously directed yourself to do so. You would always lace your fingers the first way because this is your habit. So in essence, Weird and Different is what you experience when you are out of your habit and your comfort zone, and because of that you feel wrong and discombobulated.

So now you see how habit dictates your actions. We do the same things over and over again because they feel right to us. What if what you feel is right is actually wrong? Recognizing when the wrong is just Weird and Different gives you a tool to recognize habit and the information to con-sciously redirect your activity.

Furniture certainly does not help us to sit well. First off, you really need a hard chair underneath you to get the feedback to locate the sitz bones. Even if the chair is firm, the level of the seat is very important, too. Chairs that have backward-sloping seats should be avoided. You find these chairs in many schools, auditoriums, and cinemas.

We need a chair revolution in this world. Such a simple thing would change the high rate of back and neck pain.

Something else to consider is a sitting wedge. They come in varying heights and density. Your hips want to be higher or lower than your knees.

When you see someone sitting in a full squat, they are comfortable be-cause their hips are lower than their knees. Most of us who come from a Western culture cannot sit like this. A sitting wedge will lift your hips a little higher than your knees and thus make sitting more comfortable. I like the inflatable Gymnic Movin'. Because it is inflatable, it is easy to take with you, and you can determine its density when you blow it up.

Another very important piece of information is this: do not sit in one position for more than twenty to thirty minutes. Our bodies are designed to move, not to sit still. If we sit still for any length of time, we start to stiffen up. So if you have a task like working at the computer, writing, or doing crafts or gardening or anything that requires you to stay in one position for any duration, you need to shift your position. All you have to do is stand up and sit down. Perhaps you can walk across the room. Just change your position. Set a timer as a reminder for every thirty minutes. This simple change will make you less stiff, reduce pain, and make your task much more enjoyable.

Some of my students lament the fact that they just spent an enormous amount of money on an ergonomic office chair only to have me tell them that the best thing for them would be a fifty-dollar wedge and a kitchen chair picked up at a local garage sale for five dollars. Also, think twice about having wheels on your office chair. The mobility of the chair could force you to brace your knees and hips to prevent from rolling too much.

If you have no other option than to sit on soft furniture like a couch or easy chair, use pillows to support your back and bring you forward onto your sitz bones.

http://mderbyshire.com/your-guided-sitting-practice/

We have covered a lot of ground in this first lesson. Let me summarize what we have learned and what you can practice now.

- First find a hard chair, like a kitchen or dining-room chair.
- Sit toward the front edge of the chair, and slide your hands under your bum, palms up. Find your sitz bones, and slide your hands out.
- Place your feet underneath you.
- Think about your head on top of your spine. With your hands, locate your AO joint. Think about softening your neck, your tongue, and your jaw.
- Think about your spine releasing away from your pelvis in the direction of your head.
- Do not try to sit up straight.
- Continue to think of yourself in this way.
- Pay attention to yourself whenever you sit.

Notice that you have not been asked to do anything. You have only been asked to think about yourself. Because the mind and the body are one, when we affect the body, we affect the mind, and when we affect the mind, we affect the body. You are you; your body and your mind are completely interconnected. Our new and improved way of thinking about ourselves changes our well-being—physical and mental.

Throughout your learning you will constantly bump into Weird and Different. Essentially this means that what you think you are doing or feeling isn't necessarily what you are actually doing or feeling. So often what feels right to you only feels that way because it is what you are accustomed to. It is your habit, but it is not necessarily right.

You are now learning a whole new way to think about yourself, and it is thinking in these new directions that will bring about enormous changes.

CHAPTER 3

Get Up, Stand Up

> You are, at this moment, standing right in the
> middle of your own acres of diamonds.
> —EARL NIGHTINGALE

When talking about driving an SUV in a New England snowstorm, one of my brothers likes to say, "They may have four-wheel drive, but do they have four-wheel stop?" I often think how this statement applies to our daily lives. Most of us are terrific at the doing, but we are really bad at the stopping. Doing defines our culture. Trying hard also defines us. If at first you don't succeed, try, try again, and make sure that you try harder. To do and to try go hand in hand. In elementary school, we even got a grade for it: A for effort!

When a person comes to me for a lesson, my first instruction is, "Do not help me." This always elicits a laugh. We like being in control. We are hardwired to help, to be ready, to be on our guard, to try, and to try harder. And now with smartphones and iPads, we are expected to stay tuned in to the media, our jobs, our families, and our friends twenty-four seven. We live in a go-go world, when what we really need is to stop.

Observation of our habit is the first step, and stopping is the second step. As my good friend and colleague Pamela Blanc likes to say, "We cannot change what we do not know. Once we know our habit(s), we can choose to stop them." In order to change, we need to stop the habit. Stopping is paramount to letting go of a habit. If we do not stop the original habit, then we would just be piling habit on top of habit.

This ability to stop is a skill. It is a conscious way for you to stop responding in a habitual way. Alexander used the word *inhibition* to describe this ability to stop. *Inhibition* here does not have the negative connotation that Freud gave it.

An example of inhibition that most can relate to is if someone cut you off while driving. Your immediate reaction might be to gesticulate wildly, but when you inhibit, you wait to respond. The waiting gives you time to decide how to respond. The waiting gives you the opportunity to choose. Choice eliminates the habitual response. So instead of being incited to road rage, you may just wave at the offending driver. The stopping gives you the time and the space to make a decision. Do you want to be rude, or do you want to make your point in a friendly way?

Inhibition is mindfulness. It is mindfully stopping your habitual response so that you can consciously decide if you would like to do something else. When you inhibit, you really have choice!

Today you are going to learn how to choose to go from sitting to standing in a more efficient way! Take a seat on your hard kitchen or dining-room chair. Let's start by stopping. Just stop and wait and tell yourself that you are here and present. Let's use what we learned in the previous chapter. By now you know to sit on your sitz bones with your feet underneath you. You have a better understanding of where your head is in relation to your spine. You know not to try but instead to think. You are going to think about your head on top of your spine and your spine expanding away from your pelvis toward your head.

Let me add some more instruction. Think about your tongue and your jaw. When it comes to the relationship of your head and your spine, your tongue is a very important muscle. Surely you know that your tongue rests in your mouth, but did you know it goes all the way back to your throat and connects to the hyoid bone? If you place two hands on either side of your jaw and trace your jaw toward your throat, you will locate your hyoid bone.

The tongue is the most flexible muscle in the body and is incredibly strong. When your tongue is tense, your neck will be tense, and when your neck is tense, your head will not be resting easily on top of the spine.

You will know that your tongue is tense when it is stuck to the roof of your mouth! The good thing is that you can consciously redirect your tongue to release. So try this sitting in your new way. Tell yourself to soften your tongue. Tell yourself to soften the tip of the tongue and the middle and the back of the tongue that goes all the way into your throat. What do you notice?

Some of you might notice that the head drops slightly forward.

The reason that the head may drop forward is because the front of the head is heavier than the back of the head. When your tongue and thus your neck are contracted, your neck and back muscles pull your head back and down. When your tongue and your neck are released, your head may automatically fall forward in a very subtle way.

Remember Alexander's enormous observation back in the 1890s that the relationship of the head to the rest of the spine influences functioning. With time and practice, your tongue will release and eventually lay at the bottom of your mouth more consistently. And by practice I don't mean trying hard; I mean attention. Attending to your tongue is a practice, just as meditating is a practice. Make your practice easy. An easy practice is repetition that cultivates joy!

http://mderbyshire.com/**dont-clench-your-jaw**/

Now let's talk about the muscles of the jaw. Clenching your jaw and grinding your teeth are signs of excessive and unnecessary stress and contribute to TMJ and other afflictions of the jaw, teeth, and sinuses.

When you are sitting and standing and moving well without undue strain, your teeth should not be touching. Your teeth should only be touching when you are eating (or maybe if you are angry). You have upper teeth that are connected to your skull, and you have lower teeth that are connected to your jaw. The jaw acts like a hinge, and when it is released, it will drop down away from the skull and the upper teeth.

When you are superrelaxed—for instance, when you fall asleep in an armchair—your jaw will drop down and back toward your throat.

Let's go back to your chair and sit in your new and improved way with your Guided Sitting instructions. Think about your head on top of the spine and the location of the atlanto-occipital joint. Now turn your head from side to side. Has your head's range of motion improved?

Let's do the opposite: clench your teeth, and move your head right and left. The clenching of the jaw probably limits the head's range of motion. Conventional wisdom would tell you that if you wanted to increase the range of motion of any part of your body, you would need to stretch and strain. Instead of stretching, you have improved your range of motion by consciously thinking of not clenching your jaw. It is that simple.

Some people carry a tremendous amount of strain in their eyes, and this, too, can impede head rotation. If releasing the jaw did not improve head movement, then think of softening your eyes. Staring is a sure sign of eyestrain and holding. Staring narrows your field of vision.

Allow yourself to look and notice your peripheral vision. Think of your eyes as softening and your peripheral vision as expanding. As if floating, allow your eyes to look to the right. Thinking of your Guided Sitting instructions—stop and wait, allowing the neck, tongue, and jaw to soften, head on top of the spine, and spine releasing up—gently turn your head to the right. Do the same to the left side.

As we age, head mobility can become compromised. A daily practice of turning your head from side to side in such a way will ensure a healthy range of motion!

You may be wondering why all this tongue tightening and jaw clenching is so important. Remember, the way your head relates to the rest of your spine determines how well you move. It has a direct correlation with how balanced, mobile, and agile you are. And this is not coming just from me; there have been studies to prove it. In 1999 and 2008, two research studies were conducted involving AT and balance in seniors. The first measured improvements in Functional Reach (Dennis 1999), which is an assessment of balance. This study was essentially about flexibility. The second measured improvement in activities found in the Fullerton Advanced Balance Scale (Batson and Barker 2010), which is a series of movement-based activities used by physical therapists to assess the risk of falling. So in other words, they researched AT and mobility. These studies support the concept that AT improves balance by improving flexibility and mobility.

http://mderbyshire.com/**feet-too-far-forward**/

Let's go back to our chair because now we are going to play around with standing. Place your feet in front of you, not under you as instructed before. Now try to stand up. What happened? It is much more difficult to stand up in this way with your feet too far in front of you. Do it again in the same way, and notice what happens with your head and neck. Your chin juts forward, and your head is pulled back and down. Standing like this ensures poor use.

Remember, we do not want to distort the head/neck/spine relationship. We want to allow the head to rest on top of the spine as much as possible. Now bring your feet underneath you, and sit on your sitz bones. Stop and wait and think about the Guided Sitting Instructions. Allow your nose to drop just a bit and stand up. Was that different? Was it easier? If it was not easier, perhaps you are interfering in one of the following ways.

- You are getting up too soon, which means that you are not waiting for your weight to go over your feet, and thus you are standing up while on your heels. Wait a moment more before you stand so that your weight is distributed over the arch of your foot.
- You are still stiffening and contracting your neck and tongue and jaw and thus pulling your head back and down. Tell yourself that standing does not need a lot of effort. Tell yourself that standing is easy. Rethink your original instructions of softening the neck, the tongue, and the jaw, and allow your nose to drop a tiny bit and stand again.

http://mderbyshire.com/easy-standing/

- You are pushing your feet and legs into the ground. You do not need to push to stand up. This idea is astonishing to most people.

To demonstrate this, take your hands and place them palm to palm in front of your chest. Now press your hands together and notice their resistance. This is how you are standing now. This is way too difficult—no wonder it is hard to get out of the chair and onto your feet! Now place your hands palm to palm again, and lightly and gently move your hands back and forth. This is how your feet should meet the floor. Just let your feet meet the floor to stand. Do not push.

http://mderbyshire.com/dont-push-with-your-feet-to-stand/

- You are lifting your feet up off the floor before you stand. Leave your feet alone. Just let them meet the floor. Remember, it is not important that your whole foot be on the floor—just some of the foot needs to be touching.
- You have a preconceived idea that standing takes a lot of physical effort. Tell yourself that you are not going to stand. Go to stand, and before you get onto your feet, stop. Notice how much effort you are bringing to stand. Tell yourself that you are going to stand with half that effort. Go to stand and stop. Again cut your effort in half. Now go to stand, and see how little effort it really takes. You are refining your standing by making it easier.

http://mderbyshire.com/**make-standing-easier-still**/

- You are going for the gold! What? Yes, going for the gold is when you want the outcome, the results, and the finish line, but you are not paying attention to the way in which you get there. When you go for the gold, or *endgain* as Alexnader called it, you bypass process. Here, your process is to stop and pay attention to yourself and release unnecessary tension. When you go for the gold, you just get more and more tense trying to reach your goal. Going for the gold is a very helpful concept. When approaching any task, it is convenient and effective to ask yourself, am I going for the gold here? If you find that you are, then change your approach.

Now that you are on your feet, it is time to sit down. Reorganize yourself before you sit. This is what you are doing when you stop and think about your head on top of your spine. You are reorganizing yourself when you think about softening your neck, your tongue, and your jaw so that the head and spine are better coordinated and the spine can release up toward your head.

Think about your shoulders. Think of your shoulders as moving away from each other, right shoulder expanding toward the right wall and left shoulder expanding toward the left wall.

Notice where you place your feet. Most people stand with their feet far too close. Your feet should be roughly about shoulder-width apart.

Continue to give yourself the instructions to not tighten your neck so that the head springs a little forward and up. Remember, *forward* means just drop your nose slightly. Now, bending your ankles, knees, and hips all at the same time...sit in the chair.

Make sure you are folding at your hip joints. Your hips are the largest joints in your body. They are designed to lower and raise you, so use them!

Most people have no idea where their hips are actually located. If you were to put your hands on your hips, you are actually placing your hands on the top of the pelvis called the iliac crest. Your hips are located roughly a couple of inches from either side of your pubic bone. This is the point of articulation for your hip.

If you have the habit of not folding at the hip in order to sit and stand, then there is a very good chance that when you start to do just that, you will feel as if you are sticking your bum out! Remember, this is Weird and Different, and you are not sticking your bum out—it just feels that way. Watch yourself in the mirror to make sure that you are folding at your ankles, knees, and hips.

When you stand and when you sit, your knees should track forward and down. You don't want your knees to pull inward, nor do you want your legs to splay outward. If you have the habit of pulling your knees inward toward each other, tell yourself to wait and think of your knees as directing straight forward from the hip. If you have the opposite tendency of splaying your knees out, then think of them also directing forward. Slowly these habits will change, but it takes attention.

You may be wondering why I repeat the same instructions over and over again. This is how we learn. We learn through repetition and reinforcement. There is no place else where you will be told to stop, wait, and soften your neck, tongue, and jaw. There is no place where this will be reinforced. Think of me as your softening coach. This new way of thinking about yourself should be repeated over and over again in an easy and joyful practice.

A good way to reinforce these instructions is to place Post-it notes in strategic spots around your house, car, and anywhere you spend a lot of time. Place the notes in places where you naturally stop, such as the bath-room mirror, the coffee maker, the computer, the car, any workplace, and any doorway and place that you make a transition. The Post-it notes will remind you to think these new thoughts and thus help you change from moving with strain and stiffness to a new you, moving with balance, agility, and ease!

You have certainly been building on your skills in lesson 2! Bravo! Please humor my repetition. You will see that the first half of the summary is a rep-etition of the last chapter. These are your building blocks. This is your new mantra. Thinking like this is your new litany. I love this quote by Zig Ziglar, "Repetition is the mother of learning, the father of action, which makes it the architect of accomplishment!"

- First find a hard chair, like a kitchen or dining-room chair.
- Sit toward the front edge of the chair, and slide your hands under your bum cheeks, palms up. Find your sitz bones, and slide your hands out.
- Place your feet underneath you.
- Think about your head on top of your spine. With your hands, lo-cate your AO joint. Think about softening your neck, your tongue, and your jaw.
- Think about your spine releasing away from your pelvis in the direc-tion of your head.
- Do not try to sit up straight.
- Continue to think of yourself in this way.
- Ask yourself if you are going for the gold.
- Without tightening your neck, stand up.
- Think about your head on top of your spine. With your hands, lo-cate your AO joint. Think about softening your neck, your tongue, and your jaw.
- Think about your spine aiming away from your pelvis in the direc-tion of your head.

- Do not try to stand up straight.
- Continue to think of yourself in this way.
- Allow your shoulders to release away from each other.
- Notice where your feet are, and place them about shoulder-width apart.

CHAPTER 4

Stand by Me

I have a confidence about my life that comes
from standing tall on my own two feet.
—JANE FONDA

As we age, our ability to maintain balance—that is, keeping the body's mass over the feet—can become an enormous concern. As was stated earlier, the Centers for Disease Control and Prevention (CDC) says that medical costs for seniors' falls are $34 billion annually. The CDC also says that one out of three seniors fall every year. Every year at least 250,000 of these falls result in a hip fracture, and 20 percent of these people will die in one year. Those who survive typically need extensive help with daily tasks. Yes, these numbers are worrisome. But simple remedies exist that can improve and maintain balance and help prevent falls.

The feet are incredibly complex, with twenty-eight bones, thirty-three joints, and more than one hundred tendons, muscles, and ligaments. They are probably the most maligned parts of the body. Frequently squeezed into ill-fitting shoes, they are squashed and deformed and forgotten until pain strikes. Not only can foot pain be unbearable, but it also disrupts how you stand and walk, causing other aches and pains.

The first thing that most people can do to improve the situation is to buy shoes a half or a full size bigger than usual. Years ago, one would go to the shoe store and be properly fitted for a pair of shoes. Today most of us buy the shoes off the rack with no real understanding of shoe fit. Your toes need to be able to release forward from the foot. If the shoe is too short, this will not be possible.

Shoes with thick or inflexible soles cause other problems. Your foot is amazingly flexible, and when it makes contact with the ground, it needs to be able to express that flexibility. If the sole of the shoe prevents this movement either because it is too stiff or too thick, your balance is compromised.

High heels are a disaster and should be worn only for special occasions...if ever. There are a lot of good shoemakers making sensible shoes. Investing in well-fitting, flexible shoes should be a top priority!

The foot has three arches: the medial arch, the lateral arch, and the medial-longitudinal arch. The medial-longitudinal arch is big and is the most recognizable.

Let's think about this arch as if it were a trampoline. If you were to jump on a trampoline and you wanted to stay in one spot while jumping, you would make yourself very stiff and rigid. But if you were happy to jump all over the trampoline, then you would let yourself be less tense, and you would be able to jump all around the surface of the trampoline.

By now you know what to think about rigidity and stiffness in the body. This large arch is like a trampoline, and it provides an ample amount of area for you to shift your weight.

Most of us stand with our feet too close together and with our weight back on our heels. Standing on your heels is like putting on the parking brake. When we subtly shift our weight forward over the large arch, we take off the parking brake and are ready for movement and are better balanced.

Please stand on your feet. If you have a tendency to lose your balance, then put the back of a chair in front of you for safety.

http://mderbyshire.com/**wafting-and-waving**/

Our next activity is called Wafting and Waving. Just as with sitting you start with your Guided Sitting Instructions, so, too, with standing, you will start with your Guided Standing Instructions. Tell yourself to stop, wait, and let go of your tongue, jaw, and neck. Think of your spine springing toward your head. Allow yourself to gently shift your weight over the large arch. Gently trace a circle with your weight over both of your feet. Start with your weight mostly on one foot, and then shift your weight to the other foot. And do this so that your whole body is swaying in a circular pattern. Do this for a few rotations, and then change direction. Notice if there are spots where your weight does not want to go.

Gently encourage yourself to explore those spots. Shift your weight back and forth from foot to foot. Do you notice how much movement your foot is capable of supporting?

Now try the Rocking Activity. Shift your weight to your heels, and then shift your weight over your arch. Notice that when poised over your arch, you are more ready and available to move.

You can learn so much about your habitual patterns of tension with both of these activities. For instance, does your weight tend to favor one foot? When you shift your weight toward your toes, do you feel that you are too far forward? Could this "too far forward" feeling be weird and different, meaning you feel too far forward, only because you habitually stand on your heels?

When you shift your weight from foot to foot, can you find your plumb line? Are there other things you are noticing? Think about athletes such as tennis players or martial artists. They are over their arches and ready to move!

This seemingly subtle shift will make your standing and your walking better balanced and more dynamic. Do this Wafting and Waving and Rocking Activity daily to encourage more flexible and responsive feet to stand on.

Standing in one place can be very difficult and taxing. Standing in line at the bank or the grocery store or any other place is the perfect place for you to practice Wafting and Waving. You will find that this little movement will make standing easier.

Another way for you to make standing more efficient is to think of yourself as standing on your skeleton rather than using your muscles to hold you up. Think of this: your skeleton supports you, and your muscles move you.

Culturally we have this misconception that if we were only stronger, we would move better. I am not saying that strength is not important, but I am saying it is less important than you think. Once again, think about small children. They don't do squats with forty pounds on their shoulders, and yet they are able to run and play all day. Allow yourself to stand on your bones, and allow the bones to support all of you. Tell yourself that your muscles are not girding or bracing to hold you up.

So now that you have played around with where you place your weight over your feet, it is time for your Guided Standing Practice. Stand on your feet, and place your feet about shoulder-width apart. Discover the resilient large arch. Think about softening your neck, tongue, and jaw so that the head can release forward and the spine can spring up, allowing for a widening and lengthening of the back. Allow your shoulders to expand away from each other. Tell yourself to release your bum muscles—so many of us tighten our bums. This is unnecessary muscular tension. You do not need it!

Notice your knees. Many people overstraighten their knees by pushing the knee toward the back. Your knee can do one of two things: it can be pushed back or not. Make sure that you are not pushing your knee backward, and if you are, let it go. I'm not asking you to bend the knee. I am just asking that you do not push it backward.

Think about your feet, and allow the toes to release forward from the heel. Allow the toes to soften and to lengthen.

Then gently repeat these instructions without judgment. Think of yourself in a gentle and expansive way. Notice where you are holding onto unnecessary tension, and let it go.

There is another way for you to stand that will make standing more comfortable. It is a position that you probably know very well. It is the squat!

http://mderbyshire.com/powerful-standing/

Stand with your feet about shoulder-width apart, and think about the Guided Standing Instructions. (Stop and wait. Let go of unnecessary tension in your neck, tongue, and jaw, and think about your shoulders expanding away from each other. Think about your spine springing toward your head. Think about your head releasing forward and up.) Remember, these are thoughts. You are not trying to do anything. You are just thinking these thoughts. Notice how easily you are standing.

Now bend at your ankles, knees, and hips as if you are going to sit down, but don't. Lower yourself a few inches. This is the squat. The importance of the squat is recognized in all sports. Baseball, football, and tennis players, golfers, runners, and even equestrians use this position to start. You can use the squat when you wash dishes, cook, brush your teeth, or do the laundry.

Most of us when doing these chores have a tendency to belly up to the bar, meaning that we sink in our hips and push our stomachs forward. This puts enormous undue strain on our backs and our necks. The squat frees up your back and neck and makes movement easier.

Let's talk a little bit about anatomy. You have two types of skeletal muscles (muscles used to support and move your skeleton): postural muscles and phasic muscles. Your postural muscles include spinal muscles, some of your abdominal muscles, hip flexors, and calf muscles. These muscles are composed primarily of slow-twitch muscle fibers and are designed to work all day long, maintaining your posture. Some of your phasic muscles are the gluteals, the abdominal wall, the triceps, the biceps, and the trapezius. The phasic muscles are composed mostly of fast-twitch fibers and are designed for short spurts of work. A good way to think of it is that your postural muscles support you, and your phasic muscles move you.

When you have good use, your postural muscles fire first and support the movement of the phasic muscles. But if your use is not good, the postural muscles are not recruited and therefore are not supporting the phasic muscles (Garlick 1991). Poor use shortens postural muscles and limits their mobility, and this affects strength. Good use does the opposite and lengthens postural muscles. So, in short, you are getting a workout just by using yourself well.

The things that you have learned so far, like sitting on your sitz bones, your head releasing off the top of your spine, your feet underneath you while you sit, standing over your arch, and the squat are all ways in which you are improving your use, allowing your body to move in ways you are designed to move. Of course, the squat will not answer all of your needs. For instance, it would be less efficient to vacuum the floor in a squat.

I would like to introduce another effective position, the lunge. The lunge is a dynamic way for you to move and perform a task in an efficient and effortless way.

http://mderbyshire.com/better-standing-the-lunge/

Start with your feet roughly shoulder-width apart. Stop and wait and attend to yourself by thinking of your Guided Standing Instructions. Place one foot forward onto the floor, all the while thinking of your spine aiming toward your head and your head releasing forward and up. You should be bending at the hip, not at your waist. You can shift your weight forward onto your front foot, or you can have equal weight on both feet. The lunge makes many activities easier—anything that requires pushing, pulling, or even picking something up off the floor. The main thing with the squat and lunge is that you are bending at your ankles, knees, and hips.

The hips are the largest joints in your body. They are designed to lower and raise you. Your waist is not a joint. In fact, your waist is not an anatomical term! The waist is an area of the body defined by fashion designers! Nature did not design you to bend at the waist, so make it easy and bend at the hips, knees, and ankles.

As you continue to learn how to use yourself more efficiently, it is essential to remember that you cannot apply effort to your activities. Words like *effort*, *try*, *force*, and *exert* are not constructive when thinking about yourself.

http://mderbyshire.com/lets-lighten-up/

Here's a simple illustration: Make a fist with one of your hands. Let it go, and release your hand. Now make a fist again, and let that go. Now, ever so gently, make the shape of a fist with your hand, but don't clinch it; just hold it gently in the shape of a fist.

Here is my point: You have a preconceived idea of what a fist is and the amount of effort that it takes to make a fist. The first two fists that you made were most certainly strong and tight. The gentle, loose fist is still a fist, but it is very different from the first two. The fist is like your day, your life, and all that you do. We have a preconceived idea (habit) regarding what it means to live our days and our lives, just as we do regarding how to make a fist.

Most of us bring far too much muscular tension to whatever we do. We have a preconceived idea as to what this might be. What if we approached life a little like the gentle fist? It would still be your life. You would still get things done.

What if you let go of the grind and the trying and the effort? You will still have your intention, and your intention will get you where you want to be. Your trying just gets in the way. Your trying only emphasizes what you already know. It emphasizes your habits and your poor use. It is better to stop trying; let go and lighten up. When you stop trying, you will find that you will move more easily. We just feel better when we move more easily.

Lesson 3 was full of valuable information. This is what you learned:

- Don't try. Let go and lighten up.
- Wear bigger shoes that are thin soled and flexible.
- Review your Guided Standing Practice:
  1. Stand on your feet, and place your feet about shoulder-width apart.
  2. Discover the resilient large arch.
  3. Think about softening your neck, tongue, and jaw so that the head can release forward and the spine can release up, allowing for a widening and lengthening of the back.
  4. Allow your shoulders to release away from each other. Tell yourself to let go of your bum muscles.
  5. Make sure that you are not pushing your knees backward, and if you are, let them go.
  6. Think about your feet and allow the toes to release forward from the foot. Allow the toes to soften and to lengthen.
  7. Gently repeat these instructions without judgment. Think of yourself in a gentle and expansive way.
  8. Notice where you are holding onto unnecessary tension and release it.
- *Wafting and Waving Activity.* Recite your Guided Standing Practice to yourself. Start to shift your weight on your feet. Start to draw a circle on your feet with your weight.
- *Rocking Activity.* Recite the above directions to yourself. Rock your body from your heal forward to the large arch.
- *Squat.* Stop and wait. Stand with your feet roughly shoulder-width apart. Recite the Guided Standing Practice. While thinking up with your spine and head, allow yourself to bend at the ankles, knees, and hips.
- *Lunge.* This is the same as above, bu this time step forward with one foot.

CHAPTER 5

Let It Be

There is more to life than increasing its speed.
—Mahatma Gandhi

I f you were told that there is a daily practice that requires you to carve out fifteen to twenty minutes of your day, and in exchange it would decrease or eliminate neuromuscular pain, improve your energy level, calm your anxiety, clear your head, and make you just feel better all over, would you do it? The Alexander Technique Lie-Down, sometimes referred to Semisupine, provides all of these benefits and more. To learn this practice is to stop the habit of busyness. To learn how to stop, wait, and decide how to react as opposed to habitually and unconsciously responding is a skill that can be learned, practiced, and improved.

Very few things in life are linear. Life is more like a spiral. You never know when something that you have learned in your past will become relevant or useful. The AT practice of lying down in semisupine position is like that. How can a simple practice done fifteen to twenty minutes once or twice a day completely transform one's life over time?

In order for us to change, we do not need to move one hundred and eighty degrees. One just needs to move a few degrees from one's position to set off in a different direction. The daily practice of the AT Lie-Down is a way in which to move those few degrees.

http://mderbyshire.com/at-lie-down/

To practice the AT Lie-Down, you will want to get down onto the floor. If this is challenging for you, then do not hesitate to use a chair to assist you. If you are unable to get down to the floor, then you may do your AT Lie-Down in a bed, but be sure to use books behind your head instead of a pillow.

Find a spot on the floor with carpeting or a rug. You can use a yoga mat or a blanket if you would like. You want a firm surface to lie on.

Place a short stack of paperback books on the floor. Start with a stack roughly two inches high. This is where you will place your head. Then add or subtract books as necessary for the height to feel comfortable. You do not want so many books that you tuck your chin or have too few books so that your head falls back onto the books. Paperback books are the best. Hardback books are too hard and uncomfortable. If you find that even paperback books are too uncomfortable, then place a facecloth or small towel on top. This should provide enough of a cushion to make it more comfortable.

Sit on the floor with your back to the books and with your knees bent. Lower your chin to your chest, and roll down through your back until your head rests on the books. You may use your arms and hands to assist you. When you get onto the floor, your head should be resting on the books.

- Place your hands on your rib cage with your elbows pointing away from your sides.
- Place your feet so that they are flat and your knees are pointing up to the ceiling.

- Your feet should be close to your bum at a comfortable distance.
- If you find that your legs begin to tire or shake, then ask yourself to release the tension in your legs. You may also lower one leg so that it is long and on the floor. Lie this way for fifteen to twenty minutes one or two times a day.

The book height is not a science. It may change throughout your lie-down, and it may change every day from lie-down to lie-down. The books should not touch your neck but simply support your head so your neck can release.

Although the AT Lie-Down is relaxing, this is not a meditation. Keep your eyes open. You may find similarities between this position and some meditation or yoga practices, but the difference with AT is the way in which you think about yourself. You are changing the way you think about yourself and giving yourself specific instructions on how to be.

While lying there, think about allowing yourself to be on the floor and allowing your head to rest on the books. Don't press yourself into the floor. Just let yourself be on the floor.

- Think of your spine expanding from your tailbone and your pelvis in the direction of your head.
- Think of softening and letting go of the tension in your neck.
- Think of your head resting on the books and your neck, tongue, and jaw unclenching.
- Think of your shoulders expanding away from each other.
- Think of your knees releasing toward the ceiling.
- Think of your toes expanding away from your heels.
- Notice any place where you may be holding on to tension, and ask yourself to let go of that tension.
- If your lower back feels tight, just lift your pelvis in a pelvic tilt, and lower your back to the floor.
- If you have trouble or strain keeping your knees up, then you can place your lower legs on a chair.

- If you have pain in your lower back, placing your lower legs on a chair is also very effective and can alleviate pain. Bring the chair close to your bum so that the legs are fully supported. Some people will feel tightness, stiffness, or even pain when they first start the AT Lie-Down practice. If this is your experience, then start off with shorter periods and gradually work yourself up to the full fifteen to twenty minutes.

http://mderbyshire.com/**lie-down-with-your-legs-on-a-chair**/

The Alexander Technique is like a toolbox for life. Among your tools you have *inhibition* and *direction*. Inhibition provides you with the space and time to reset yourself and choose to react or not, and direction allows you to consciously expand your psychophysical self. You have Weird and Different that allows you to assess habit and the changing of habit. The concept of going for the gold gives you a way to identify when you have strayed from the process to the results. The AT Lie-Down is another very important tool. It, too, is another way to reset, but it also provides rest. As said before, we live in a go-go world, and we need to know how to stop. The AT Lie-Down teaches you how to stop.

You may find at first that you are too restless to lie down for twenty minutes. That is OK. You can start with five minutes and gradually add more time. Soon you will be amazed at how much you enjoy lying on the floor for a full twenty minutes. This is time for you! This is time for you to reset. This is similar to unplugging the computer when it needs to reset. You can "unplug" yourself to reset and reorganize yourself.

There are many physiological changes that happen while on the floor. Have you ever heard the adage that you are taller in the morning than you are at night? This is true! You are about one inch taller when you wake up after a night's sleep. As the day goes on, the cartilage between your vertebral discs gets compressed. Gravity and your activity compress the cartilage. When you lie down to go to sleep, the cartilage regains its original level and thus increases your height. The AT Lie-Down gives the cartilage another opportunity to restore itself and for your spine to return to optimum length.

The practice of lying down also calms your nervous system, clears your head, and helps you to become less reactive. It gives you space and time to observe yourself so that you can notice where you are holding excessive muscular tension.

Lying down also gives your muscles time to reset to their resting length. Because we all have a tendency to brace ourselves and to perch, lying down gives us the opportunity to consciously let go of tension throughout our system. It gives you the opportunity to key into your senses so that you may return to the moment.

Lying down is such a simple activity, and yet it brings enormous rewards and change. Embrace this! Incorporate it into your day. If there is nothing else that you take away from this book, it is this: set aside the fifteen to twenty minutes every day to lie down in semisupine position, with your head on some books. Notice habitual patterns of tension, be they physical or mental, and ask yourself to let these go. Self-care is health care. Taking care of yourself must be a top priority.

While lying down you may listen to some quiet music, but do not watch TV or talk on the phone or look at your iPad or even have a conversation with a loved one or friend. This is your time to calm your system. It will surprise you how these communications can rev you up and distract you from yourself and the purpose of lying down. No distractions—just you, the books, and the floor.

Once you have become proficient at lying down, one interesting way to approach it is to think about something that may be somewhat upsetting. Notice how you tense up. Now continue to have that thought, but attend to yourself by not tightening your neck, tongue, and jaw. Notice the floor underneath you, and let go of your head and your back. Has the upsetting thought changed in any way?

When we affect the physical, we affect the mental, and when we affect the mental, we affect the physical. This is what is meant by the psycho-physical. We have mind-body unity. Paying attention to how you use yourself calms the body and the mind. Just letting go of physical tension while thinking a challenging thought can soften the sharpness of the emotion.

http://mderbyshire.com/how-to-get-off-the-floor/

The way in which you get up off the floor is just as important as how you get down onto the floor and how you practice the AT Lie-Down. Decide whether you want to get up on your right side or your left side. Now stop and wait and tell yourself that this is not about getting up but rather about releasing old habits of muscular tension. Wait. Release. Now turn your eyes in the chosen direction, and gently turn your head. Lower the leg on this side so it is resting on the floor. Press the foot of the opposite leg into the floor, and bring yourself onto your side, turning your shoulders and pelvis. You should now be lying in a fetal position. Using your top arm and hand, press your hand onto the floor, and bring yourself to a sitting position. Next, bring yourself onto all fours to stand up. If standing up is difficult, you should use the nearby chair to assist you.

http://mderbyshire.com/use-a-chair-to-help-you-to-stand/

Now that you are on your feet, notice if you feel any different. Notice your demeanor. Notice your back and your shoulders. Where is your head? How are your feet? Are you feeling lighter, easier, freer? Notice the language being used to describe you! Every word is about stopping and releasing and expanding. Your words and language are your thoughts, and they matter.

http://mderbyshire.com/cement/

Let's play a game that I learned from my colleague Nancy Romita. You can do this with yourself, but it works even better with a partner. One of you is partner A, and the other is partner B. Both of you are standing up.

Partner A, put your arms around partner B, and try to move or lift him or her. Notice that you are able to move partner B.

Next, partner A, recite this script to partner B:

"Imagine there is giant hole at the top of your head, and into this hole is poured wet, gray cement. This wet, gray cement is filling up your skull, traveling down through your neck and into your lungs and chest. This wet, gray, heavy cement is filling up your abdomen and pelvis. Heavy, wet cement is pouring through your thighs, knees, and lower leg. This heavy, gray cement is moving into the ankles and feet. Heavy, gray cement is surrounding the foot."

Partner A then tries to move or pick up partner B. Partner A cannot move partner B. Partner B is so heavy that he or she actually feels as if he or she were full of cement.

We don't want to leave partner B in the quagmire of cement, so let's lighten him or her up. Partner A, recite this script:

"You are standing in a pool of water, and the water is fresh and clean and sparkly. Allow the sparkly water to fill your feet and move through your ankles. This bright, sparkly water is swelling through your lower leg and up into your thighs. Allow this fresh water to fill up your abdomen and move into your lungs and chest. This bright, sparkly water is swelling up into your throat and your skull and is bubbling out through the crown of your head." Now, partner A, try to lift partner B! Ta-da! It is so easy to move partner A.

Do you see the power of language and how your words and thus your thoughts affect your physicality? There is scientific evidence that this is true. Neuroscientist and Alexander Technique teacher Rajal Cohen did a study using the phrase *lighten up* to see how it would affect posture, movement, and balance. Rajal runs the Mind in Movement Laboratory at the University of Idaho, where her work is "inspired by the idea that cognitive factors are important for controlling action." In this study her subjects were people with Parkinson's disease. Parkinson's is known for causing, among other things, rigid muscles, unsteady stance, and poor control of movement. Dr. Cohen found that when she asked these people to think about "lightening up," (rather than "pulling up" or "relaxing") their torsos became less rigid, their stance became steadier, and they were able to initiate movement more smoothly, indicating better control (Cohen 2015).

The cement game we just played demonstrates the importance of choosing language that benefits you. What old tapes are going through your head? What words do you use that just pull you down and compress you? Language is so important. Expressions like *try harder; double down; no pain, no gain*; and *pull yourself up by the bootstraps* are not constructive or helpful. We need language that is kinder and gentler. This game illustrates how simple it can be. So choose *lighten up* or *allow, free up* or *let go*. Your psychophysical self will thank you!

AT Lie-Down Summary

1. Find a spot on the floor with carpeting or a rug.
2. Place a pile of paperback books on the floor. This is where you will place your head.
3. Sit in front of the books. Lower your chin to your chest, and roll down so that your head rests on the books. You should not have so many books that you tuck your chin or have too few books so that your head falls back onto the books. The book height is not a science. It may change throughout your lie-down, and it may change from lie-down to lie-down.
4. Place your hands on your ribs. Place your feet so that they are flat and your knees are pointing up to the ceiling. You may place the

back of your legs on a chair seat, if you prefer. Bring the chair close to your bum.

5. Think about yourself lying this way. Think about allowing your head to release onto the books. Think about your neck being soft and free. Think about releasing tension in your tongue and jaw. Think about allowing the spine to release away from the pelvis in the direction of the head. Think about allowing your back to release onto the floor as well as the soles of your feet and your elbows. Think about allowing your shoulders to release away from each other. Allow your elbows to release away from your shoulders. Allow the wrist to release away from the elbow. Allow the fingers to release away from the palms. Think about allowing your knees to release toward the ceiling. Allow the thigh to release up and the shin to release up. Think about your heel releasing back and down from the foot and the toes releasing forward from the heel. Just think these thoughts; don't try to do them.

6. Lie this way for fifteen to twenty minutes one or two times a day.

CHAPTER 6

Every Breath You Take

Remember to breathe. It is, after all, the secret of life.
—GREGORY MAGUIRE, *A LION AMONG MEN*

Exhale. Close your mouth and wait. Wait some more, and wait a little longer. Now let the air come in through your nose. Wait and then exhale. Close your mouth and wait, wait some more, and wait a little longer. Now let the air come in through your nose. Wait and then exhale. Close your mouth and wait, wait some more, and wait a little longer. Now let the air come in through your nose. Return to breathing normally. Notice how much calmer you are. Let us proceed.

There is nothing like your breath. Obviously, you can't live without it. It sustains you. It feeds oxygen to your muscles and removes carbon dioxide from your body. It gives you voice. Without it, you cannot whisper, hum, speak, sing, or whistle.

Breathing is responsive. Every emotion elicits a different kind of breath. It expresses a gasp, a sigh, a laugh, a chuckle, or a growl. Breathing is primal. We do it all day and all night, unconscious of its presence. Yet we can, for short periods of time, alter its rhythm. We can speed it up, and we can slow it down. We can take deep breaths, or we can take shallow breaths. We can run, and our breathing speeds up, too, staying with us and helping us to perform this challenging task. Breathing has the potential to be transformative. Breathing is like a chameleon, changing with every aspect of your life. But just as poor use compromises your mobility, poor use also compromises your breathing.

Breathing is movement, too. The rhythmic expansion and release of the rib cage needs to be free of restrictions in order to provide you with the optimal amount of oxygen to support your activity. The tightening and clenching of your neck, tongue, and jaw will tighten your rib cage, diaphragm, and abdomen, and each of these is essential to breathing.

When you are moving well, your breathing will be free and unrestricted. Your rib cage and diaphragm will move in a synchronized way. And although we breathe all day long, it is typically not something that we give much consideration. Let's change that. Let's give it some consideration! There are many myths and misconceptions about breathing. In this chapter we will briefly look at the physiology of breathing, how poor use affects your breath, and the Alexander Technique way of approaching breath that will improve oxygen intake and reduce anxiety.

A healthy adult at rest takes between twelve and twenty breaths per minute. Of course, this rate will increase with physical activity. You have two lungs—a right lung and a left lung—that sit on either side of your heart. The lungs and heart are enclosed by your ribs.

A large, flat muscle called the diaphragm is attached to the lower ribs and separates the thoracic cavity from the abdomen. There are two phases to breathing: inhalation or inspiration and exhalation. Inhalation is when the oxygen comes in through the mouth or nose and goes into the lungs, from where it is absorbed into the bloodstream. When you inhale, the diaphragm descends while air enters the lungs, and the ribs expand outward.

The ribs have the potential to expand in many directions. For instance, you may know that when you inhale, the top of the rib cage rises, but did you know that the ribs in your back can expand as well? A common misconception is that the lungs are only in the front part of the chest, but, in fact, your lungs also reside in your back. So your back also has the potential to expand and contract with each breath. Just bringing your awareness to this fact will deepen and expand your breathing.

Another misunderstanding is what is known as belly breathing or dia-phragmatic breathing. This misnomer is important because we do not ac-tually breathe into our bellies or our diaphragm. We breathe into our lungs, and the movement of the diaphragm downward increases the volume of the thorax and moves the ribs, thus allowing more room for the expanding lungs. The confusion arises because as the diaphragm descends, it pushes down on the viscera in the abdomen, and in turn, the abdomen moves out-ward. Obviously you cannot breathe into your belly; you breathe into your lungs. A lot of unnecessary tension is created when you try to take a deep breath to expand your belly.

The second phase, exhalation, is when you expel carbon dioxide. When you exhale, the diaphragm releases up toward the lungs, sending air out, and the ribs respond. Inhalation and exhalation are reminiscent of waves lapping on the shore. The exhalation is like the wave advancing onto the beach, and the inhalation is the wave's retreat.

Breathing is a powerful tool that when called upon can have a profound effect on your mood and stress and anxiety levels. We started this chapter with a very simple breathing exercise that within seconds may have calmed you down. This breathing exercise began with the exhalation.

Slow breathing stimulates your parasympathetic nervous system that is responsible for, among other things, slowing your heart rate, lowering your blood pressure, and increasing digestive and intestinal activity. In contrast, rapid and shallow breathing is controlled by the sympathetic nervous sys-tem, which is associated with the fight-or-flight response.

Slow breathing releases the hormones oxytocin and prolactin (other-wise known as the love hormones), which make you feel good. Slow breath-ing also depresses the stress hormone cortisol. Pay attention to your breath in response to the following list of words: *anxious, nervous, sad, relaxed, difficult, scary,* and *angry.* Did your breathing change?

You know that when you are in a tense situation, you hold your breath, and you have to remind yourself to breathe. Now observe how your breath-ing is affected with these words: *happy, blissful, serene, delight,* and *content-ed.* Emotions affect breathing, and conversely, breathing affects emotions!

How wonderful is that! All you need to calm yourself down, improve your situation, relieve tension, and make you feel better is all around you, and it is free! Exhale, and let breathing oxygen happen!

Let's try some activities that will demonstrate how improved use affects your breathing. Sit on your hard chair, and slump or slouch. Look at yourself in the mirror. Take a breath. Notice how difficult it is to breathe? When slumped and compressed like this, how can you ever expect to breathe well? There is little room for air and little room for the movement of your lungs, ribs, or diaphragm.

Come back to sitting on your sitz bones, feet underneath you, softening your neck, tongue, and jaw, and allowing your spine to spring toward your head. Take a breath. Notice now how much easier it is to breathe.

Many of us have been told that in order to maintain good posture, we need to suck in our guts or abdomen. Well, let's do just that. Suck in your stomach. Now take a breath. Once again it is impossible to take a satisfactory breath. Do you see now how unnecessary muscular tension interferes with this most essential act?

The saying "The road to hell is paved with good intentions" is one of my favorite expressions. There is so much we do to ourselves that, although well intentioned, is just plain harmful. Sucking in your stomach or your gut does nothing to improve posture. It only interferes with your breathing.

http://mderbyshire.com/exhale-and-wait-to-breathe/

Let's set up an experiment. Organize yourself with your new guiding instructions. Take a deep breath, and then exhale. You probably noticed quite a bit of tension in your upper chest while inhaling. Some people have remarked to me that they feel a little claustrophobic when inhaling like this.

Let's do the opposite and exhale, and then wait and wait some more. Allow your breath to come in through your nose and mouth but only when you feel the need. You are not trying to hold your breath; instead, you are waiting for an impulse for the breath to occur.

Exhale, close your mouth, and wait. Wait some more, and wait a little longer. Now let the air come in through your nose. Wait and then exhale. Close your mouth and wait, wait some more, and wait a little longer. Now let the air come in through your nose. Wait and then exhale. Close your mouth and wait, wait some more, and wait a little longer. Now let the air come in through your nose. Return to breathing normally. This is our easy-breathing practice. I call it Exhale and Wait to Breathe.

Did you notice any changes when breathing this way? Were there any changes in your rib expansion? The strongest side of breathing's retreat and advance is the advance or inhalation of the oxygen.

Most certainly, we all tried as little kids to hold our breaths in a fit of rage only to be succumbed by one gigantic inhalation. One can only hold one's breath for so long, and then nature takes over and fills us with oxygen. Exhaling first, waiting, and allowing the air to flow is calming, restorative, and freeing! So don't take a breath; let the breath take you!

Exhale and Wait to Breathe is a powerful, stress-busting, anxiety-stopping, and mood-enhancing tool. If someone has made you angry, then bring an Exhale and Wait to Breathe to the rescue! Stuck in traffic and late for an appointment? Exhale and Wait to Breathe. Is the nurse about to take your blood pressure? You can lower it with Exhale and Wait to Breathe. If you are having trouble falling asleep, then try five to eight repetitions of Exhale and Wait to Breathe, and you can get rid of counting sheep. If you are afraid to speak in public, then pull up Exhale and Wait to Breathe, and fear no more! It works. There are no side effects, and it is free.

You are learning easy, effective ways to improve your health. Better use means better functioning, and better functioning means a healthier you with better balance, breathing, movement, and life. Self-care is health care! Exhale and Wait to Breathe is another thing you can add to your practice that will improve your being.

Breathing Summary. Exhale and Wait to Breathe.

Let us make this as simple as can be.

1. Exhale. You can exhale with a whispered "ah" sound or any vowel sound. Make it easy.
2. Close your lips. Wait. Wait some more. And wait a little while longer.
3. Allow the air to come in through the nostrils. Wait a moment. Exhale.
4. Close your lips. Wait. Wait some more. And wait a little while longer.
5. Allow the air to come in through the nostrils. Wait a moment.
6. Close your lips. Wait. Wait some more. And wait a little while longer.
7. Allow the air to come in through the nostrils. Wait a moment.
8. You can do as many of these as you like. If you get light headed from all the oxygen, then stop. Breathe normally.

CHAPTER 7

Walk This Way

An early-morning walk is a blessing for the whole day.
—HENRY DAVID THOREAU

Have you ever heard that walking is "controlled falling"? When you walk well, your head leads the movement and your foot comes forward to prevent you from falling on the ground. Imagine a child first learning how to walk.

Most adults shift their weight from side to side when they walk. If you were to exaggerate this movement, it would look like a waddle, but if you watch a child walk, they walk forward and straight. Children don't waddle.

One problem with the waddle is that you lose the momentum that each step generates. It's as if you are applying a brake with each step. Instead, if you think of yourself walking forward and not side to side, you will discover that your legs and feet will dynamically flow underneath you. Walking dynamically with forward intention will make walking easier and more efficient.

Another problem with the waddle is that the foot doesn't articulate with the ground in a dynamic way, thus having an undesirable effect on balance and stride. When your foot works well, it strikes the ground slightly to the outside and to the front of the heel. Your weight then crosses the large arch, the medial-longitudinal arch, over to the big toe.

Your big toe has two very important jobs. It helps you balance, and it propels you forward. Many adults do not engage the big toe at all. Instead, they hold the toe up and only walk on the soles of their feet. This inevitably results in the side-to-side waddle. People who do this to an extreme will create holes with their big toes on the tops of their sneakers and slippers.

http://mderbyshire.com/**dynamic-walk**/

If you were to exaggerate this movement, you would eventually shuffle. The good news is that if you are shuffling now, with a little conscious thought, you can stop shuffling and move into a dynamic walk.

Remember, shoes that fit well with a pliable and thin sole are essential for happy feet and dynamic walking. Stay away from bulky, padded sneakers that, although comfortable, are not flexible. Your toes need to be able to splay as you move. Your feet need to flex and adjust in order to keep you balanced. Make sure that your shoes are large enough to accommodate this movement. Also, overly tight socks can impede movement and diminish balance.

If you are unsteady on your feet or you fear falling, hiking poles are a great way to ensure balance and gain confidence. Whether you use one or two poles is up to you, but the added point of contact is a huge benefit. Used by hikers and climbers worldwide, the hiking pole is lightweight yet sturdy. The pole height is adjustable, and it comes with a strap that goes around your wrist. To customize the height, hold your forearms at a right angle from your upper arm. You can purchase hiking poles at many sporting-goods stores.

Let's practice walking.

Our first step is always to stop and wait. Think of your Guided Standing Instructions. (Soften your tongue, your jaw, and your neck. Allow the spine to spring away from the pelvis toward the head. Allow the head to release forward and up so that the nose may drop slightly.) Thinking up and forward, look ahead with the intention of walking toward something in front of you.

Now take a step, and then continue walking. Tell yourself to walk through the big toe. Allow your knees to release forward. What do you notice? When you are walking well, you should feel as if you are floating. Your feet may feel as if they are rolling along the floor. You may feel light and buoyant, and you should feel propelled forward.

Next add the arms. When you walk well, your arms should swing by your side. Arm swinging improves stability and reduces the amount of energy used while walking. And here is a little bit of trivia—when runners want to increase their speed, they are told to move their arms faster, not their legs! So swinging your arms is important when going out for a walk.

When your left foot comes forward, your right arm should come forward and vice versa. This is called cross patterning. Most of us cross pattern. When children crawl, they practice cross patterning by bringing the opposite leg forward with the opposing arm. The cross-pattern movement creates a pathway between the left and right sides of the brain. This is one reason why it is so important for children to crawl; they learn coordination through cross patterning.

Cognitive issues such as dyslexia have been linked to an inability to cross pattern well. It has been my experience working with seniors that many lose the ability to cross pattern or swing their arms in opposition to their legs, and thus their coordination suffers. The good news is that you can encourage and relearn how to cross pattern. Let's try it!

http://mderbyshire.com/**cross-patterning**/

I call this next sequence Wait, Shift, and Turn. Take your hard chair, and sit on your sitz bones. Think of your Guided Sitting instructions (stop and wait and release your tongue, neck, and jaw so that your head can release forward and up). Now shift your weight over to your right sitz bone. Continue to think light and easy, and continue to attend to yourself. Now shift your left shoulder forward. Keep your head looking forward. Return to neutral; by that, I mean come back to sitting over both sitz bones with your shoulders squared. Next, do the opposite. Shift your weight over your left sitz bone. While attending to your directions, bring your right shoulder forward while keeping your head looking forward, and return to neutral.

Do several of these Wait, Shift, and Turn sequences. Notice that it is as if you are walking on your sitz bones. I always feel as if I am in the Broadway musical *West Side Story*, singing "When You're a Jet," when I do this! This simple sequence helps to restore latent cross patterning.

Now stand up and walk, and notice how much easier it is to swing the opposite arm to the opposite leg. If cross patterning is difficult for you, commit yourself to practice this daily. Eventually you will improve the swinging of your arms as well as your balance and coordination.

http://mderbyshire.com/**watch-your-elbows**/

A common position seniors adopt that interferes with their walking is leaning forward from the waist or upper back. In order to counterbalance their weight being so far forward, they bend their elbows and hold them up and back behind themselves. Look at yourself in your mirror, and see if this is you. Just by looking at this position, you can see how your balance is compromised. People in this position are often told to "stand up straight," and so they haul themselves up through the torso and shove their shoulders back, but as we all know all too well, this never works. Let's approach this habit another way.

As always, stop and wait and give yourself your Guided Standing Instructions, and ask yourself to lower your elbows toward your waist and allow the arms to come forward and down. While you do this, ask yourself to allow the spine to spring up toward your head.

Because you have brought about a lot of change, you are most certainly going to be experiencing Weird and Different. You are going to feel wrong, and you are probably going to feel that you are standing too far back. This is only in contrast to the fact that you were too far forward.

Has your breathing improved with this shift? Are you more upright? What is your head-neck relationship like? The release of your arms by your side provides a nice bit of direction up through the spine.

Now take a walk, and allow your arms to swing. Here is something else to think about. Think about where you are coming from, not what you are going toward. Think about what you are leaving behind you as you walk. This thought will allow you to walk taller.

Because the forward stance has become habituated, it is going to take a lot of attention and easy practice to reorganize yourself with your elbows forward and down and your spine lengthening up toward your skull.

Most of us have a dominant leg when we walk and stand. Usually it is the leg that we start off with. It is probably the leg that you always use when you start to climb stairs. Sometimes it will be the leg that you lean on. Because this leg is the first to be engaged, it is also the leg that will be overly tense. A simple way for you to spread the workload is to count up to three as you walk. Each stride will take one count. In this way, you will alternate the burden of the starting leg.

We all need to walk and walk more. Our culture is far too sedentary. I am not saying anything new, but if you don't walk, you won't be able to walk. I have a saying that goes like this: "If you do it, you can do it, but if you don't do it, you can't." It may seem obvious, but it never is. If you want to walk, then you need to walk. If you have not been walking much, it is never too late to start walking more.

The human body is designed to move. We are sitting ourselves to death. We need to walk every single day. Use walking sticks, and set realistic goals for yourself. You may start by walking to your mailbox and back. Increase the distance in increments. Do not overextend yourself. Add a few minutes at a time. When you increase your distance, wait a few days before increasing again.

Give your body time to develop strength and endurance. If you find yourself getting tired, then lessen your walking time for a few days. Your body responds to new challenges by becoming stronger. This is what exercise is all about. Challenge builds strength. But the challenge has to be appropriate. A goal of thirty minutes of walking a day may seem daunting at first, but by gradually increasing your time, soon it will become a reality.

Walking on different surfaces will also add a new level of challenge. Think about it—most of the surfaces we walk on are hard and flat, such as flooring in your home or the pavement in your driveway or sidewalk. But we humans are designed to walk on grass, rocks, sand, and dirt. These surfaces are rough and not uniformly even. In short, pavement does not challenge you. If you don't live in a large city, you can easily add some rough surfaces to your walking practice. So grab your walking sticks, and head out onto some grass or gravel!

We have spent time talking about how to walk, so now let's talk about why we walk. This is the point in the book where we take all that we learned about improving how you function and then make sure that you use your new and improved functioning in a way that will have profound impacts on your health.

There are two things I want you to embrace. Walking is exercise, and exercise is movement. Don't sell walking short. This is my soapbox. There is a whole fitness industry that wants to make you believe that you need this or that piece of exercise equipment or you need to be subscribing to this or that form of exercise in order to be effective. The result is that a lot of people are really intimidated by all the hoopla. If you have a body and are reasonably mobile, you can move. Even if you are unsteady on your feet, you can still explore movement sitting on your hard chair.

You have learned many new skills. You have learned how to organize yourself in a way so that movement is easier. In particular, walking is easier and is more efficient. Set aside time in your day to go for a walk and think about yourself in this new and improved way while walking. This is mindfulness. Constructively paying attention to yourself is the way in which you will improve the way you move and react. Wear thinly soled flexible shoes. Stay away from heavily padded sneakers. Increase your walking in increments of a few minutes, and space out the increments every few days. Use walking sticks to help with balance. Walk on uneven surfaces to challenge and improve balance and mobility. Count to three while walking so as to ensure an even and consistent gait. Make walking a daily activity.

- Stop, wait, and tell yourself to release tension in your jaw, tongue, and neck.
- While freeing your neck, allow your head to release forward and up off the top of the spine.
- Allow your back to lengthen and widen. Remember, you are not doing anything; you are thinking these thoughts only.
- Thinking up to go forward, look and see what you want to walk toward. Now take a step, and continue walking.
- Remember to think that you are walking through the big toe.
- Allow the knee to release forward.
- Allow the arms to swing, opposite arm to opposite leg.
- Start a daily walking practice. Increase time in increments, and slowly work up to thirty minutes a day.

CHAPTER 8

Let's Get Physical

> Get out in the day.
> —FRANK KENNEDY

The one thing that will improve the quality of your life and health is consistent exercise or movement. Movement is crucial for our well-being.

The benefits of exercise/movement are impressive. Exercise improves heart, lung, and circulatory systems, reduces body fat, regulates the digestive system, improves glucose tolerance and insulin resistance, regulates your sleep cycle, lowers your cholesterol, increases blood supply to your muscles, increases the threshold for muscle fatigue, reduces anxiety and depression, reverses aging, and makes you happy. There is no doubt that exercise/movement heals.

This is where the Alexander Technique plays a crucial role. Everything that you have learned from this book up to this point has been talking about how you move. Everything before now has addressed the way in which you move. The quality of your movement is paramount.

How can you ever be expected to exercise if you cannot move more easily or without pain?

Here is the answer, loud and clear. Before you set out to exercise and while you exercise, be it going for a walk or starting a tennis game, you apply the technique. You stop and wait and tell yourself to soften your tongue, neck, and jaw and to think of your spine releasing toward your head. You think of yourself in an expansive way, and then you proceed with your walk or your tennis. You periodically check in with yourself, and you go through the same self-instruction. You are mindfully instructing yourself how to move in a freeing way.

Think of it this way. If you were to watch Yo-Yo Ma play the cello, he wouldn't just walk on stage, sit down, and play his cello. He would sit down, stop, and reorganize himself before he was to play his cello.

We all should be doing a similar thing as we go through our day, whether it is washing dishes or running a marathon. We all need to be stopping and reorganizing ourselves so that the quality of our movement and being is addressed and thus improved.

This is mindful movement, and I promise you that when you start to approach your exercise with your mind, then the drudgery that some feel toward exercise will vanish. You will become so fascinated by how your thoughts improve your experience that a whole new world will open up to you. You will feel more integrated and better connected with yourself.

We humans were designed to move, yet everything in our culture is asking for us to sit. According to Galen Cranz, author of the book *The Chair*, chairs are a relative newcomer to our culture (Cranz 2000). For common people, chairs did not exist until about two hundred years ago. Those who owned chairs were very wealthy and powerful; think of the throne.

Before that, people would sit on a log or a stool, or they would squat. Many cultures today still don't use chairs, and instead they squat. It wasn't until the Industrial Revolution that furniture became available to the masses, and it wasn't until the huge developments in the textile industry that stuffed furniture became ubiquitous.

By the Victorian era (1837–1901), furniture was stuffed and padded in ways never before imaginable. Before this, one might have rested on a stool or log or squatted on his or her haunches, but now the temptation to spend hours sitting in an overstuffed chair has become too much.

Our once-standing and moving culture has become a sitting and lounging one, and our bodies and minds do not like it. Here are some pointers as to how to navigate our sitting culture.

- When it's available, always choose a hard chair, like a kitchen or dining-room chair. This also applies to the chair you use for your computer or crafts. You do not need an expensive "ergonomic" office chair. Do not waste your money. You can find inexpensive hard chairs in many department stores, or better yet, recycle and pick one up at a local yard sale.
- Sit on a sitting wedge. Your hips like to be higher than your knees, and a conventional chair typically has your hips and knees at the same level. If you shop online, just enter "sitting wedge," and dozens will pop up. I like the Gymnic Movin' Sit Inflatable Seat Cushion. This sitting wedge is reminiscent of a ball chair. For some, a more stable wedge would be better or preferred. Make sure that the wedge is firm. You do not want a soft wedge. You want the wedge to be at least two inches on the high side.
- We all sit on couches and soft furniture, but you should put pillows behind your back so that you are sitting on your sitz bones. If you are buying new furniture, make sure that it is not too low or too soft. Both low and soft make it incredibly difficult to get out of.
- Do not sit for too long a period of time. Stand up at least every thirty minutes. You don't even have to walk around. You can just stand up and sit down. Your body wants to move, and sitting in one position for a long period of time (thirty minutes or longer) will cause stiffness and strain and even pain.
- Choose a barstool! My joke is that everyone thinks that sitting on a barstool is easier because he or she is sitting at the bar! But no—it is easier because the barstool places your hips higher than your knees!
- If you experience strain when you are sitting in your new and improved way, that is, on your sitz bones, feet underneath you, neck,

tongue, and jaw released, head on top of the spine, and spine releasing toward your head, then bring yourself all the way to the back of the chair so that your back may lean against the chair back. Over time, you will develop the strength to sit up easily for longer periods of time.

- Choose to stand! If you are able, stand rather than sit. There are lots of standing desks now. Practice your Guided Standing (chapter 4) while working at your standing desk, or practice your guided standing while just standing.
- Bring your work to you so that you don't have to lean into your work. Your computer screen should be at eye level. Your keypad should be roughly in line with your hands and wrists or a bit lower so that your elbows are at sixty to ninety degrees. If you use a smartphone, bring the phone to you; don't look down to the phone. Articulate your head from the AO joint to look down. Do not look down with your neck. If you are reading a book, bring the book up to you. Use pillows to support your arms and the book. If you knit or crochet, bring the needlework up to you; do not bend over to do the work. This is a good way to think about it. Do not let anything disrupt the integrity of your good use. Bring your work to you.

Enough of this sitting. Let's get back to moving! Here is a movement sequence that is simple and easy, yet most effective. It is a great one to do before you get out of bed every morning and after each AT Lie-Down. I call it Your Daily Moves.

If you are like many people, the first moments when you get on your feet after a night's sleep can be very painful. Much of the problem is that we have been lying in pretty much the same position all night, and because of the lack of movement, we stiffen up. By moving a little before getting out of bed, you can alleviate the pain. Here is a sequence I call Feel Better Back.

http://mderbyshire.com/feel-better-back/

1. Lie on your back with your knees bent in a semisupine position. This is the same position you are in when you do the AT Lie-Down with your feet on the floor and your knees bent. Draw one knee toward the chest and keep the other foot on the bed. Alternate with the other knee. Do this several times. Make sure that one foot makes contact with the bed or the floor at any given time. Or you can do this on the floor after your AT Lie-Down.

2. Place both feet on the bed or the floor and drop your knees to one side and your head to the opposite side. Alternate from side to side. Do this several times.

3. Place feet wider apart, and then drop one knee toward your midline and return. Then drop the other knee toward your midline and return. Do this several times.

4. Cross one ankle over the opposite knee, and then draw your knees toward your chest. You may use your hands to guide your legs. Do this several times, and then change sides. This movement requires a good deal of flexibility. If you are unable to do this at first, do not worry; eventually you will.

5. Do all of the above moves with as little effort as possible. Make them EASY!

6. The way in which you get out of bed or off the floor is important. Don't just haul yourself up. Lengthen the leg on the side you will be turning toward. Bend the opposite leg so that the foot is on the bed or floor. Turn your eyes in the direction you are going to get up. Then turn your head. Then turn your shoulders and your waist, and with your bent leg, push yourself onto your side. Press your top hand into the bed or floor, and gently push yourself into a sitting position.

We all have what I refer to as our Movement Vocabulary. Our bodies move in a certain way. For instance, our knees and elbows act as hinges, and our ankles have all sorts of ways to articulate, as do our hips. The potential is there for us to move in many different ways, but they are specific ways.

When we were kids, we ran, hopped, tumbled, and jumped, exploring this movement vocabulary, but as we age and because of our sedentary culture, this vocabulary becomes very limited. Our movement expression is diminished. In addition, this Movement Vocabulary has a Range of Motion. Your Range of Motion is demonstrated when you try to reach for something or try to take a bigger step or put on a shirt. It is how far you can reach or extend your limbs or turn your head or torso.

So two very important aspects of our movement can lessen as we age—our Movement Vocabulary and our Range of Motion. The amazing and wonderful thing is that if you have lost the ability to move in a certain way with a limited ability to extend and reach, you can regain these abilities.

As I've said, one of my mantras goes like this; if you do it, you can do it; if you don't do it, you can't. In order to be able to move, you have to move. This may seem so obvious, but as we age, we have a very real tendency to shrink our Movement Vocabulary and decrease our Range of Motion. We need to be doing the exact opposite. The phrase "use it or lose it" is absolutely correct. So let's use it, so we don't lose it. And if we feel that we have "lost it," then let's regain it! It can be done!

Below, you will find four very simple movements or patterns of movements that you can practice every day. They are designed to address your Movement Vocabulary, agility, and Range of Motion. Consider them a warm-up for your daily activities.

As you have just learned in this book, you need to practice every task, even the difficult task, with ease and joy. In Christopher McDougall's book *Born to Run*, he discovers that the secret to running a hundred miles a day in sweltering heat by the Tarahumara Indians of Mexico's Copper Canyon is that they do it joyfully. They do not approach running as drudgery but as a joyful expression of play and communication. Let's follow their lead and find joy in our movement and in our being. Join me in having fun!

The Long-Highway Look

http://mderbyshire.com/**long-highway-look**/

Using your hard chair, sit in your new and improved way. Be sure to be on your sitz bones. Place your feet underneath you. Think of your Guided Instructions. Notice where your head and neck and spine articulate. Turn your head to the right. Return to center. Turn your head to the left. Make this easy. If you have difficulty turning your head (and for some, this is a very real concern), lead the movement with your eyes. Allow your eyes to shift to the right. Make sure that it is just your eyes moving and not your head. Most people will turn their heads when asked to shift their eyes left or right. So stop, soften, and allow just your eyes to turn right, and then easily allow your head to follow. Do not try to force the movement. Do the same to the left. The practice of turning your head side to side in an easy way will increase mobility.

2. Balancing Ankles

http://mderbyshire.com/**balancing-ankles**/

http://mderbyshire.com/**movemor-with-cate-reade**/

Good balance is dependent on healthy ankle mobility. Remain in your chair, and organize yourself in your new and improved way. Here is a list of movements created by my friend and colleague Cate Reade. Cate invented the MoveMor Lower Body Trainer, an ingenious yet simple piece of equipment that "helps seniors regain strength and mobility...for better physical function and falls reduction."[1] Cate's website is http://www.resistancedynamics.com/team/.

- Lift and lower your toes.
- Lift and lower your heels.
- Alternate lifting and lowering toes, with one foot and then the other.
- Rotate the toes inward and then outward.
- For pronation, roll ankles in so that your arches move downward.
- For supination, roll ankles out so that your arches lift upward.
- Make a clockwise circle with your foot, and then make a counter-clockwise circle with your foot.

In 2010 Dr. Eyal Lederman published a paper titled "The Myth of Core Stability." In it, he challenges the common belief that back pain is deterred by strong abdominal muscles. He goes so far as to say that perhaps we should do the opposite: "Maybe our patients should be encouraged to relax their trunk muscles, rather than hold them rigid?" This certainly fits in with the Alexander Technique approach. Think of small children just learning to walk. They get up on their feet, and in no time they are running around in all sorts of ways. They do not have any back pain. They did not spend time doing abdominal crunches or planks, yet they have the strength and stamina to run, jump, and play. So perhaps we should take another approach and rethink core strength.

---

1 http://www.resistancedynamics.com/product/movemor-lower-body-trainer/

3. A Healthy Back / Supple Back

http://mderbyshire.com/**a-healthy-back-is-a-supple-back**/

Here is a movement I learned from two wonderful Alexander Technique teachers, Joan and Alex Murray. I call it Healthy Back / Supple Back. Again using your chair, on your sitz bones, wait and give yourself your Guided Instructions.

- Place the backs of your hands on your thighs so that your palms are facing up.
- Allow your eyes to look down toward your chest.
- Let your head follow your eyes.
- Allow your spine to create a C shape with your back releasing behind you.
- Let your head roll down toward your lap to a comfortable position. Do not force this. If you cannot go very far, that is fine. Over time, with easy repetition, your range of motion will improve.
- If you can go further, do so. You will find that your torso will move toward your knees. Allow your palms to remain under your shoulders. Your hands will need to slide toward your knees. If you cannot go any further, then stop here.
- Those of you who are finding this easy, continue and let your head and arms drop in front of your knees. If your hands cannot reach the

floor, and this is most likely, then place your hands on your shins, ankles, or the tops of your feet. This is really important. Support allows for release. In other words, do not hang there unsupported. Your hands need to rest somewhere.

- Allow your head to hang. You will feel a wonderful passive release through the spine.
- Now just look up with your eyes toward your eyebrows. This is important. Just move your eyes and not your head.
- Now let your head follow your eyes and look straight ahead.
- Without changing the angle of the head and neck, come to a sitting position so that you are looking up toward the ceiling.
- Now easily right your head so that you are looking straight ahead.
- Easily and joyfully repeat two more times.

4. Balance Challenge

Balance also falls under the "use it or lose it" category. If you don't challenge it, it will decline. Remember, most of us are way too sedentary, and sitting down does not challenge your balance. In Scott McCredie's book *Balance*, he even suggests that our society is having more and more balance problems due to the fact that we, for the most part, only walk on hard, even surfaces such as tarmac and cement. We need to walk on uneven surfaces, such as grass and dirt roads. What is amazing and fortunate, however, is that very quickly your balance can improve. Let's do some balance activities. Use your kitchen counter or the back of your hard chair to provide support in case you need it. Your vision is one of the three systems that contribute to your balance. So where you place your eyes determines the level of difficulty. Looking down at the floor (and, of course, articulating your head at the AO joint) is the easiest. Looking straight ahead is more difficult, and closing your eyes is very difficult.

http://mderbyshire.com/**balance-with-little-foot/**

http://mderbyshire.com/**balance-with-big-foot/**

Little Foot, Big Foot. Think of your guiding instructions. Make sure that your feet are under your shoulders and not too close together. Stand on one leg. Switch to the other leg.

Walk the Plank. Place one foot in front of the other to walk forward. Do this backward.

http://mderbyshire.com/**walk-the-plank**/

Semicircle. Draw a semicircle with one foot on the floor. Do this forward and backward. Now lift the foot off the floor, and see if you can do the same thing. You can tap your foot along the floor as you draw the semicircle. Do the same with the other leg.

http://mderbyshire.com/**the-semi-circle**/

Lateral Lift. Lift your leg to the side and off the floor. Do the same to the other side.

Movin' and Groovin'

http://mderbyshire.com/movin-and-groovin/

http://mderbyshire.com/**over-over**/

http://mderbyshire.com/**heel-toe**/

About FM Alexander

Frederick Matthias Alexander (FM, as he liked to be called) was an actor born in Tasmania, Australia, in 1869. He grew up on a large farm surrounded by animals, particularly horses. He was a keen observer of nature, especially how humans and animals moved. However, he was a sickly child and was asthmatic. Because of his health, he could not attend school with other children and was tutored at home. His tutor passed on to Alexander a passion for Shakespeare.

In his early twenties, Alexander moved to Sydney to start an acting career. In Sydney in the 1890s, it was very popular for actors to recite long passages of Shakespeare. Alexander became a well-respected actor, but the breathing issues that plagued him as a child were now jeopardizing his career. Alexander had developed laryngitis. His voice would become hoarse during his performance. His friends and colleagues reported that they could hear him gasp for breath while on stage. This was well before the time of amplified sound and microphones. Alexander knew that it would be the end of his career if he could not solve his vocal problems. He sought the help of medical doctors and was told to rest his voice. This helped to a certain extent, but when he got back on stage, he would once again become hoarse. It was at this point that Alexander realized that it was something that he was *doing* that was bringing about his hoarseness, since when he rested and stopped *doing*, his voice would improve.

He was determined to find out what this doing was. Using a mirror, he watched himself speak with an "indoor" voice. Then he observed himself while reciting and "projecting" as if he was on stage. Eventually he was able to detect three habits that were present when he spoke normally, which became more pronounced when he went to recite.

The first habit was "sucking in air." The second habit was what he described as "depressing his larynx." The third and most important habit was "pulling his head back and down."

He tried to stop these habits. No matter how hard he tried, he could not prevent the first two habits. Eventually he focused on the third habit, pulling the head back and down. He found that he was able to prevent this habit, and to his astonishment, the other two habits disappeared!

Alexander then realized that the relationship of the head, the neck, and the spine acts as a coordinating mechanism for the entire body. If the relationship of the head and the neck is poorly coordinated, the functioning of the whole is poorly coordinated as well.

Alexander's improved voice and breathing brought other actors and singers to him for instruction. His reputation grew, and he was known as the Breathing Man. Soon people realized that not only did their voices improve but also that other aches and pains disappeared as well. At the urging of a friend in the medical community, Alexander moved to London in 1904 to bring his observations to a wider audience. He spent the rest of his life improving his technique.

He was highly respected in London and worked with many influential people of the time. The famous educator and philosopher John Dewey was a student of his, as well as the author Aldous Huxley and the playwright George Bernard Shaw. He wrote four books providing insights on the development and application of the Alexander Technique: *Man's Supreme Inheritance, The Use of the Self, Constructive Conscious Control of the Individual*, and *The Universal Constant in Living*.

Several scientific studies have validated the technique, including an extensive study conducted by the *British Medical Journal* that concluded

"Lessons in the Alexander technique offer an individualized approach designed to develop lifelong skills for self-care that help people recognize, understand, and avoid poor habits affecting postural tone and neuromuscular coordination."[2] In the prestigious *Annals of Internal Medicine*, they reported that a series of Alexander Technique lessons resulted in "statistically significant and clinically relevant long-term reductions in neck pain and disability at twelve months."[3]

Many athletes and celebrities have endorsed the technique, including Hugh Jackman, Benedict Cumberbatch, Madonna, Sting, Kevin Kline, John Cleese, Judi Dench, and Julie Andrews, to name a few. The Alexander Technique is taught worldwide at many performing arts universities, including The Royal Academy of Dramatic Arts, Yale School of Drama, Juilliard School, as well as many others.

The technique is taught worldwide. There are Alexander Technique Societies in seventeen different countries, with over three thousand member teachers.

- To find a teacher near you in the United States, contact http://www.amsatonline.org.
- To find a teacher near you in the United Kingdom, contact http://alexandertechnique.co.uk/.
- To find a teacher near you in Canada, contact http://www.canstat.ca.
- To find a teacher near you in Australia, contact http://www.austat.org.au/.

---

2 http://www.bmj.com/content/337/bmj.a884
3 http://www.annals.org/aim/article/2467961/alexander-technique-lessons-acupuncture-sessions-persons-chronic-neck-pain-randomized

Recommended Reading

Batson, Glenna, and Sarah Barker. 2010. *Studying the Efficacy of Using the Alexander Technique as Improving Balance in Healthy Elderly (Ages 62–83).* https://www.youtube.com/watch?v=INf5bGRwhZA.

Brennan, Richard. 1996. *The Alexander Technique Manual: Take control of your posture and your life*: Great Britain: Little, Brown and Company.

Cohen, Rajal G. 2015. "Lighten UP: Specific Postural Instructions Affect Axial Rigidity and Step Initiation in Patients With Parkinson Disease." nnr. sagepub.com/content/early/2015/02/09/1545968315570323.

Cranz, Galen. 2000. *The Chair: Rethinking Culture, Body, and Design*. New York: W. W. Norton & Company.

Dennis, Ron EdD. 2013. *The Posturality of the Person: A Guide to Postural Education and Therapy*. Atlanta: Posturality Press.

Dennis, Ronald, J. 1999. "Functional Reach Improvement in Normal Older Women after Alexander Technique Instruction." *Journal of Gerontology: Medical Sciences* 54A (1): M8–11.

Garlick, David George. "The Garlick Report: Muscle Fibres and Their Activation." *Direction: A Journal of the Alexander Technique* 1 (8): 6.

Langer, Ellen J. 2009. *Counterclockwise: Mindful Health and the Power of Possibility*. New York: Ballantine Books.

Gorman, David. 2014. *The Body Moveable: Blueprints of the Human Musculoskeletal System Its Structure, Mechanics, Locomotor, and Postural Functions, Sixth Edition*. Toronto: Learning Methods Publications.

Lederman, Eyal. 2008. "The Myth of Core Stability." http://www.cpdo.net/Lederman_The_myth_of_core_stability.pdf.

McCredie, Scott. 2007. *Balance: In Search of the Lost Sense*. New York: Little, Brown and Company.

McDougall, Christopher. 2009. *Born to Run: A Hidden Tribe, Superathletes, and the Greatest Race the World Has Never Seen*. New York: Alfred A. Knopf.

Reynolds, Gretchen. 2012. *The First 20 Minutes: Surprising Science Reveals How We Can Exercise Better, Train Smarter, Live Longer*. New York: Hudson Street Press.

Rootberg, Ruth. 2015. *Living the Alexander Technique: Interviews with Nine Senior Teachers*. Amherst, MA: Off the Common Books.

Vineyard, Missy. 2007. *How You Stand, How You Move, How You Live: Learning the Alexander Technique to Explore Your Mind-Body Connection and Achieve Self-Mastery*. New York: Marlowe and Company.

Vlahos, James. 2011. "Is Sitting a Lethal Activity?" *New York Times Magazine*, April 14. http://www.nytimes.com/2011/04/17/magazine/mag-17sitting-t.html.

Acknowledgments

This book was inspired by many years of teaching the Alexander Technique and fitness and movement classes. My work with seniors came through happenstance. My husband and I moved our young family to a small coastal Rhode Island town. Unbeknown to me, retirees made up a significant portion of the community. Soon my classes were full of seniors--not the young moms and dads that I had initially anticipated--and thus a whole new adventure opened up for me.

To all my students who have studied with me and have attended my classes and workshops over the years, I thank you. You taught me and were as much teachers to me as I have been for you. You know who you are. I am so blessed to have each and every one of you in my life.

To Toni Ham, Carolyn Julia Kaiser, Katharine Crellin, Linda Olsen, Bambi Truesdale Wisbach, Joan Carney, Jane McJennett, Virginia Murray, Connie Castenson, Dee Holliday, Donna Sedgwick, David Raish, Ellen Brayton, Helen Nadler, Jane Gavin, Kate Schmitt, Kathy Gardner, Nancy Chace, Norm Lofsky, Pat Dillon, Fred Burhrendorf, Suzanne St Amour, Janet Jagger, Jane Lorch, Andrea Powning, Pat Pond, George Kates, Ralph Guild, Carol Schene, Sue Cotta, David Young, Tucker Hood, Bryan Robertson, Marge Nanni, Fred and Betty Torphy, Barrett Allen, Carol Gibson, Brian LaFerte, Jerry Paquin, and Helen Woodhouse, thank you!

I would especially like to extend my heartfelt gratitude to Mike and Nancy Shand, who helped me believe that I could write this book.

Dr. Cathleen Hood, thank you for your attention and commitment to the Alexander Technique. Thank you for your encouragement to extend my reach into the medical communities. And, of course, thank you for your friendship.

To my friend and mentor, Hilary Woodhouse, your guidance, advice, and support have meant the world to me.

A huge shout-out to my Alexander Technique community. I would especially like to thank Missy Vineyard Ehrgood, Pamela Blanc, Frances Robertson, and Rajal Cohen.

To my business coach, Amira Alvarez, I could never have done this without you. Your insistence on authenticity, clarity, and purpose has been essential to me this past year.

Arif Islam is the best video editor ever, thank you!

Love and heaps of gratitude to Beverly Edwards and to all the Edwards family. We will continue to walk the beach, and we will always feel the love.

My dearest, bestest friends, Carrie Trowbridge Law, Rebecca Chace, Hilary Stevenson, Sarah Chace, Ellie Field, and Joanne Segal-Fryer, thank you.

David and Jason, you are rock stars! You too, Richard, Ralph and Peter.

Of course, thank you to my mom and dad for everything, really.

And last, but certainly not least, my family. Gordon, thank you for all of your patience teaching this Luddite mom her way around the computer. Eliza, thank you for your encouragement and insisting I be more demanding of myself. Liam, thank you for always listening and saying, "But, Mom, you can do this!"

And, of course, thank you to my beloved husband, John Petty, for always being willing to help.

Would you like to learn more?

Has this book piqued your interest? Are you recognizing that habitual patterns of emotional and muscular tension are impeding your mobility and getting in the way of your balance and confidence?

I tell my students that we are a lot like onions. We peel one layer of tension away, and voilà, there is yet another layer. Hopefully with this book, you have started to peel the first layers. But there is always more to peel.

Here's another way to think about the process. If your body is your musical instrument and you went for your first lesson to learn how to play your instrument, you would first learn the notes and then maybe a short little song like "Row, Row, Row Your Boat." And for some people just being able to play "Row, Row, Row Your Boat" may be enough. But then there are those who would like to play Chopin or Scott Joplin or Bela Bartok. If you fall into the last category, then perhaps you would like to seek out a teacher to expand your experience.

I offer unique opportunities, both in person and remotely, for you to learn how to move with better balance, agility, and ease.

I offer a personal one-on-one VIP Day where we spend an entire day figuring out your particular way of moving. You will learn how to sit better, walk better, and breathe better. I will customize movement sequences similar to those in this book that will get you moving and feeling better.

We will address activities that you engage in throughout your day, and you will learn how to do these more easily, with improved balance and agility.

I also offer a multiday experience. With a spouse or a friend, you learn all of the above, but you will also learn ways to reinforce the work with each other.

If you can't work with me in person I offer a video course by the same title as this book *Agility at Any Age*. The course is designed to further integrate what you have learned here.

Letting go of unnecessary tension is the way to free and joyful movement. Regain the confidence that you had when you were younger. Let's revolutionize aging!

Please check out my website, www.mderbyshire.com, for more details on how you can fast-track and integrate *Agility at Any Age* into your lifestyle.

http://mderbyshire.com/conclusion-thank-you-for-joining-me/

About the Author

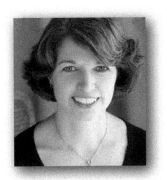

Mary Derbyshire has taught aerobics and fitness for thirty years and is certified by the American Society for the Alexander Technique (AmSAT). She has been teaching the Alexander Technique since 1995 and has taught everywhere from Dublin, Ireland, to Chicago, Illinois.

Derbyshire currently teaches in Little Compton, Rhode Island. She is passionate about helping people move easily well into their senior years.

CPSIA information can be obtained
at www.ICGtesting.com
Printed in the USA
FSHW020955290819
61537FS

9 781540 811196